Developing the Reflective Healthcare Team

Developing the Reflective Healthcare Team

Professor Tony Ghaye

C.E.O.

The International Institute of Reflective Practice, UK
and Visiting Professor at University of Wales-NEWI
and
Luleå University of Technology, Sweden

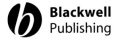
Blackwell
Publishing

© 2005 by Blackwell Publishing Ltd

Editorial offices:
Blackwell Publishing Ltd, 9600 Garsington Road, Oxford OX4 2DQ, UK
Tel: +44 (0)1865 776868
Blackwell Publishing Inc., 350 Main Street, Malden, MA 02148-5020, USA
Tel: +1 781 388 8250
Blackwell Publishing Asia Pty Ltd, 550 Swanston Street, Carlton, Victoria 3053, Australia
Tel: +61 (0)3 8359 1011

The right of the Author to be identified as the Author of this Work has been asserted in accordance with the Copyright, Designs and Patents Act 1988.

First published 2005 by Blackwell Publishing Ltd

Library of Congress Cataloging-in-Publication Data

Ghaye, Tony.
Developing the reflective healthcare team / by Tony Ghaye.
   p. ; cm.
  Includes bibliographical references and index.
  ISBN-13: 978-1-4051-0591-0 (pbk. : alk. paper)
  ISBN-10: 1-4051-0591-7 (pbk. : alk. paper)
1. Health care teams. 2. Reflection (Philosophy) 3. Learning, Psychology of.
4. Health services administration.
[DNLM: 1. Patient Care Team–organization & administration. 2. Group Processes.
3. Interprofessional Relations. 4. Problem-Based Learning. W 84.8 G411d 2005]
I. Title.

R729.5.H4G48 2005
610.69–dc22

                                                                                        2005006609
ISBN 10: 1-4051-0591-7
ISBN 13: 978-14051-0591-0

A catalogue record for this title is available from the British Library

Set in 10/12½ pt in Palatino
by SPI Publisher Services, Pondicherry, India
Printed and bound in India
by Replika Press Pvt. Ltd

The publisher's policy is to use permanent paper from mills that operate a sustainable forestry policy, and which has been manufactured from pulp processed using acid-free and elementary chlorine-free practices. Furthermore, the publisher ensures that the text paper and cover board used have met acceptable environmental accreditation standards.

For further information on Blackwell Publishing, visit our website:
www.blackwellnursing.com

Contents

Foreword

I first met Tony Ghaye in January 2004 and was impressed by his approach to developing reflective teams and reflective organisations. Being a strong advocate of reflection-in and on-practice my imagination was fired by the many approaches, developed by the international Institute of Reflective Practice-UK, to improve services rather than just focusing on individual development.

In the NHS we talk about changing cultures so that staff can better meet the health and social care needs of the population we serve. We know, however, that this takes a long time and is often ineffective if staff do not understand, or are not involved in the very changes that will develop more team-based cultures that support high quality, personalised care. This book gives us the inspiration and methods to do just this. We know that the future success of the NHS is reliant upon effective multi-disciplinary teams that can cope with ambiguity and uncertainty. By recognising the value of investing in teams to improve services, organisations can be transformed and staff will begin to think and act differently. The book offers much practical advice on how to develop more team-based working. It is therefore a 'must read' and excellent value for money.

The IRP-UK approach uses tried and tested methods to encourage better teamwork and team learning that promotes sustainable change. Does it sound too good to be true? I have personal experience of working in partnership with IRP-UK, for example on a 3 year sector-wide maternity project and also in one day workshops. The use of the approach set out in this book led to genuine innovation and real, sustainable improvement that would normally have taken longer to achieve, or perhaps been abandoned through lack of capability or capacity.

I am delighted to support the publication of this very informative text because it has much to offer health and social care professionals, managers, leaders and academics at all levels. The book captures the essence of effective teamwork. It is grounded in practice and enriched through an exploration of psychological and sociological theories that explain the complexity of team dynamics. It also clarifies different perspectives on the theory and practice of reflection, which is fundamental to understanding the value of the IRP-UK approach. It draws on a wide range of literature from a number of fields of working life. It therefore has an up-to-date and expansive feel to it. The book breaks genuinely new ground and certainly makes you think! I particularly like the chapter that introduces the reader to a new type of leader, the 'quiet leader', a concept that will appeal to those who are implementing NHS initiatives that rely on effective teamwork to make patient-led and personalised care a reality.

In part, the book acts as a toolkit to help develop reflective teams, with helpful scenarios to discuss, exercises to perform. It helps us understand how more powerful and relevant forms of reflection can be used in practice. I thought at first that the text would replace the need to contract with the Institute, but I can't emphasise enough the value of having skilled and motivated facilitators working with you and doing behind the scenes 'donkey work'. Tony Ghaye (and IRP-UK) certainly walk-the-talk.

I hope you enjoy the book. You will certainly learn from it.

Jane Marr
Formerly Director of Nursing, North West London Strategic Health
Authority
August 2005

Acknowledgements

This book has been 8 years in the making. During this time I have been deeply grateful to many people with whom I have worked. Thank you for sharing, so generously with me, your thoughts, successes and struggles in developing more reflective team-based workplace cultures. It is from your openness, your courage and commitment to improving care, through better team learning, that I have learned the most.

For providing the early encouragement and opportunity to explore team working and learning, across disciplines and workplaces, my sincere thanks go to the pioneering and inclusive work of Karen Deeny and the support offered by Linda Dunn, June Patel, Andrea Cudd, Ginny Snape, Simon Gartland, Jackie Stephen-Haynes, Pauline Wooliscroft and Sue Cuerden. I also owe a huge debt of gratitude to Gill Weale and a talented and caring group of staff particularly Rita Ridley, Bethan Stubbs, John Roberts, Angela Higgins, Maureen Webb, Linda Szaroleta, Angela Mottram, Jackie Derby and Bridget Slater.

I sincerely thank many colleagues and service users. In my conversations with them about better care through better team learning, I have come to appreciate many things. The professionalism, support and insight of Terri Wilson, Ava Gordon, Marie Tarplee, Caroline Nolan, Val Jones, David Stenson, Carol Howell, Mary Rutledge and Gwen Gerald has been much appreciated. I also wish to thank Jo Davis, Vanessa Foxall, Caroline Oliver, Ian Buchanan, Sandie Kimberley, Annette Hanny, Val Corcoran, Carole Howell, Angela Alexander, Elaine King, Heather Keating, Lorna Webley, Celia Shrimpton, Kim Probert, Ingrid Pfeiffer, Liz Vincent, Elizabeth O'Flynn, Nina Thomas and Karen Doyle. Special thanks go to Doris, Dot and a particular district nursing team.

I hope that the book suitably reflects the influence, insight and wisdom of all IRP-UK staff, Institute Members and affiliated consultants especially Nick Cripps, Sue Lillyman, Helen Gardner, Rachel Moule, Andrew Jeffrey, Sandy Nelson, Paul Wyatt, George Gregg, Ros Carnwell, Dennis Beach, Tomas Kroksmark, Eva Alerby, Maj-Lis Hörnqvist, Ed Errington, Jonathan Middleburgh, Chris Johns and John Sparrow. The on-going support of all the team at Carfax Publishing and especially Ian White, the Editorial Board and International Advisory Board members of the peer reviewed journal *Reflective Practice* is also much appreciated and is a continuous source of regeneration.

More recently I wish to acknowledge the stimulating conversations and innovative work with Jeff Lake, Pam Richards and Hamish Telfer about high performing teams, Jane Marr and Suzanne Truttero about modernizing maternity services through reflective team working, with Art Langer about the links between reflective teams, sustainable performance improvement and overall technology innovation, Russell Chalmers and The Holst Group about non-adversarial dialogue and creativity, and Mosi Kisari, Wangui Karanja and the EASUN team about the way they are undertaking excellent work with civil society organisations. Finally, I thank Robert Chambers for his inspirational work in participatory practices.

I could not have asked for a better team of staff to bring this book to fruition. My thanks go to Beth Knight and the team at Blackwell Publishing, Jules in East Africa and Kay, at IRP-UK, for their careful preparation and proof reading of the manuscript. Finally, I thank those who read and critiqued drafts of the book and to all my colleagues and family who have offered unconditional and greatly appreciated advice and moral support.

Dedication

This book is dedicated to all those teams involved in emergency care, relief, reconstruction and community rebuilding work after the tsunami disaster in December 2004, in S.E. Asia. The essence of the book is emotionally connected to, and spiritually aligned with, teams who give so generously and selflessly to others in trying to improve the livelihoods and well-being.

Part One
An Orientation to the Book

Chapter 1

The book's structure, the central question and some challenges

Structure

This is a book about meaningful learning through the practices of reflection. The purpose of this learning is to develop reflective healthcare teams that are able to sustain high quality, personalised care. After this brief orientation I describe some general starting points. These are important because the book looks at the development of reflective teams through some new and different lenses. The rest of the book is then structured in three parts (see Fig. 1.1). The first is about reflection and the practices of it. The second is about teams and how they work. The third part is about developing reflective healthcare teams through a facilitated reflective process called **TA²LK.**

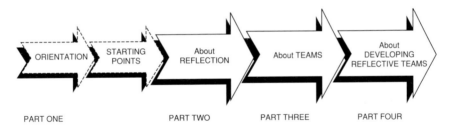

Fig 1.1   The structure of the book.

In general this book is framed by the following action-oriented question. **'How can we develop reflective healthcare teams that are able to sustain high quality, personalised care?'** In this way it responds to 'The next stage in the NHS's journey to ensure that a drive for responsive, convenient and personalised services takes root across the whole of the NHS and for all patients' (Department of Health (DoH) 2004d, p. 1). With regard to team learning and working, this book supports the much greater emphasis on developing high performing teams across the whole of the National Health Service in the UK. Fig. 1.2 shows how I begin to illuminate this question. I do so by focusing on five challenges of change. The first is the challenge of gaining and sustaining a sense that we are generally moving forwards. Without this we get stuck, practice gets outdated, we feel in a rut and go nowhere. Second is the challenge of learning through failure and how this can act as a catalyst for improving services. The third challenge is

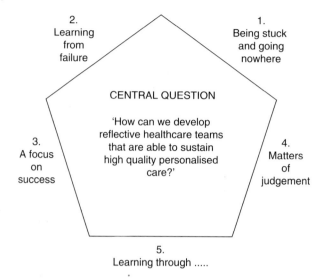

Fig 1.2   Five challenges of change.

to find ways to focus on learning from success, to notice and celebrate the successful aspects of our work, no matter how small. The fourth challenge is somewhat different. It is the challenge of making judgements about the nature, purposes, means and ends of practice. These matters embrace the notion of evidence. The fifth and final challenge is about how we might respond positively and creatively to this central question of this book, by learning through the processes of reflection.

This book is aligned with those who want even better care through improved team learning. To do this, those involved need support and a preparedness to share, reflect upon and respond positively to experiences and knowledge from a variety of sources. Three in particular are 'personal experience', 'collective knowing' and 'actionable knowledge'. The latter I define as an important synthesis of the first two. It is knowledge for improved (future) action, which we co-construct on the basis of learn-ing about what works, as well as what does not, in particular settings and circumstances. This view has a strong pragmatic and humanistic feel to it. Of necessity then, it is also about what leads to success. Knowledge alone is insufficient for service improvement. It has to be useable. Developing reflective healthcare teams requires that we find, generate and use differ-ent kinds of knowledge that have a good impact on the quality of our own and other people's working lives and on care. The book questions the notion that all knowledge belongs to 'experts', that it is always fixed rather than constantly open to refinement and that it has to be general, to be useful, rather than situated. By implication then, reflection and the various practices of it, are couched as having an interest in understanding and improving self and the actions of others, in a context. To do this, the practices of reflection have to transform personal experience and collective knowing-through-practice into publicly accessible and useable knowledge. One such use of this kind of knowledge is to sustain high quality, personalised care in particular settings.

So this is a book that goes beyond personal development. It focuses on the 'we' rather than the 'I'. The 'we' being the notion of the 'team'. Nicolini *et al.* (2004, p. 81) offer a sombre warning about the limited power of one particular, and much used, kind of reflective practice for developing teams that can transform services and workplaces. '*Individualised, private reflection is incapable of reaching and affecting the institutionalised assumptions and logic that regulates organisational action, and it is also at risk of being a sterile effort, given that individuals alone are seldom in positions to make substantial organisational changes*' However, more public forms of team (collective) reflection can only happen when they are organised (Reynolds & Vince 2004) and authorised. The process needs to be seen as legitimate and time invested in it needs to be well spent. So how can we make this happen in practice? How can we bridge the gaps between the individual, group/team and the whole organisation? I return to this later. What is important at this point is to clearly state that this book is about reflection for improved collective action not just better plans for action. Reflection is not so much valued in itself. It has to do something. It has to make a difference. It has to achieve tangible rewards to self, the team (collective) and the organisation, within certain conditions. My view on the practices of reflection is that they can enable us to 'go forwards', go further and perhaps faster, but certainly with more confidence and justification. The practices of reflection give priority to practice. What we reflect upon is that which is generated by our practice itself. It links reflective knowing with improved action, a view that needs to treat knowing seriously and sceptically. This means that we need to embrace knowing but also query it (Barnett 1996). One characteristic of the reflective team is that members acknowledge that there are many kinds of knowing that help them improve their practices. They are also aware that knowledge is partial and transient. It goes past its 'sell by date'! So knowledge about, and for, improved care needs to be constantly reviewed and put under pressure to see if it (still) helps us deliver the best for our patients and clients. Reflective teams subject themselves, their practices and the values that guide their work to planned, systematic and public scrutiny. It is fruitless therefore to try to construct a single, agreed definition of 'reflective practice'. Its meaning is to be found in the purposes of its use in particular healthcare contexts.

Being stuck and going nowhere

In responding to the book's central action-oriented question, I will be drawing upon the work of staff at the international Institute of Reflective Practice-UK, its healthcare partners and affiliated consultants during the period 1999–2004. The data base constitutes work with 753 teams in health and social care in the UK and 3211 service users. Somewhat depressingly during this period of data gathering, I have come across many teams who doubt that they can have any real and lasting influence on improving care. Sometimes this seems to be due to some genuine humility or self-doubt. Sometimes it is due to the extra work that any improvement effort requires. For others it is a consequence of two kinds of fear. First, fear that their proposed improvement will be a failure (real or imagined) and being blamed for this. Second, a fear linked with opening a floodgate of raised expectations, new possibilities and different challenges that might drown both themselves and their colleagues. So here we have the ingredients of a difficult situation on our hands. Staff end up doubting their own ability to make a difference. They end up disenchanted, disaffected and disconnected. Some 'put up and shut up', others leave the profession.

Sadly, staff within a particular healthcare organisation may know how things might be improved, but think they have no means to act, and the organisation in which they work, which would have the means to act, behaves as if it did not know. The result is impasse. Staff then behave as if investing in the status quo is the only way to survive (Rosenfeld & Tardieu 2000). So how might we get out of such an impasse? Learning through the practices of reflection gives us such an opportunity (see Part Two), but in so doing we have to get past the double-think we often get caught up in. We want change but we also want stability. We want to be responsive to others' needs but within limits. We want to develop ourselves but adopt coping strategies so that any disturbance to the ego is minimised.

Learning from failure

Many of us have a predisposition to more readily reflect on past problems and failures because these are the things we feel we need to prioritise and 'fix'. Often our encounters with technology, treatments or procedures that were 'less than hoped for', is reductionist in kind. This means we have a tendency to want to troubleshoot and fix things. In essence to break down the ambiguity, resolve any paradox, achieve more certainty and agreement, and move into the comfort zone. These 'failings' may indeed require our urgent attention. In certain circumstances this may be perfectly justified. One great influence on many of the practices of reflection reinforces this point. Dewey (1933) stated that a function of reflection is, 'to transform a situation in which there is experienced obscurity, doubt, conflict, disturbance of some sort, into a situation that is clear, coherent, settled, harmonious' (Dewey 1933, pp. 100–101). Interestingly, some (Sitkin 1996) have argued that failure stimulates a greater willingness, or readiness, to consider alternatives. It can encourage us to be more critical of current working practices. Alternatively, it can be associated with responses of denial and avoidance.

Other writers (Schein 1992) suggest that what is regarded as a failure can stimulate an 'unfreezing' process. In other words things get loosened up, un-locked and take on a different form. In turn this can initiate a new look at existing practices and policies. In healthcare there is a natural and necessary predilection for learning from failure and then turning this learning into better, safer care. Past failures and 'near misses' can be powerful catalysts for learning. The creation of the National Patient Safety Agency (NPSA) in July 2001 in the UK is a good example of this. In its remit are sustained references to improving the safety and quality of care through reporting, analysing and learning from adverse incidents and 'near misses' involving patients in the National Health Service. In essence it has reporting and learning functions, specifically learning from mistakes and problems that affect patient safety.

An essential prerequisite for becoming more proactive, rather than reactive, is the NPSA's intention to try to promote an open and fair culture in the National Health Service (NHS), encouraging all healthcare staff to report incidents without undue fear of personal reprimand. This is a cultural transformation issue where concerns like pervasive failure avoidance norms, risk aversion behaviours, self-protection, over- and under–responsibility, denial and defensiveness, have to be confronted. If we cannot be the best, the most successful at our work, then we can, at least, aspire to be the best we can. In Part Four of this book I explore the critical attributes of workplace cultures supportive of an intent to develop and sustain team learning so that we can be the best we can. I return to expressions of openness and fairness then.

A focus on success

Failures are only one kind of motivation for improving care. Another is to learn from successful and 'best' practice. The book addresses this important aspect of service improvement, specifically developing success through teams and what the constituents and conditions for this are. A central question then becomes: What constitutes success? Supportive of this are questions like: 'What does success look like?' In what ways did those involved feel that progress was being made and things were moving forwards? Like failures, successes should not be left unchallenged and certainly not unexamined, even though a dominant mindset in your workplace may well be, 'if it is not broken, then don't fiddle with it'. Success is situated in time (today's, yesterday's, last year's success) and place (in a particular speciality, in a particular hospital or community setting). It may also be limited to a particular patient or client group. Additionally, we must bear in mind that learning to learn from success is a complex, not a simple, process. For example, Sitkin (1996) suggests that success can lead to actions that preserve the status quo, an avoidance of risk taking, an over-confidence from practitioners and possibly actions where they become blind to even more effective ways of doing things. This is potentially dangerous.

Alternatively, learning from success can reaffirm both our capability and capacity for delivering and managing high quality care. Through the practices of team reflection we can learn to notice the successful aspects of our work, no matter how small, and the practical wisdom, within the team, that has led to them. This often goes unnoticed. If recorded in some way, these successes can create positive team memories. These can balance feelings derived from conversations dominated by frustration and a sense of helplessness to change things, anything, for the better. Learning to learn from reflections on success is a good preparation for learning from 'failures'. I suggest that 'troubled teams' have a tendency to be more reactive and learn in response to real performance difficulties and crises (failures). Higher performing teams have a combination of attributes that enable them to be more proactive and learn from successes as a means of 'staying sharp' and sustaining high performance. More of this in Parts Three and Four.

Matters of judgement

Success and failure are extremes. Often in our daily work 'being good enough' or 'doing the best we can in the circumstances' has to suffice. These expressions and many others like 'we did what we could' and 'this is all we could manage' occupy the ground between these two extremes and are all matters of judgement. In order to make such judgements, I suggest we need to ask ourselves three fundamental questions. They are:

1 *What are we trying to accomplish?* This helps us focus on the improvements we wish to make, on how we would like things to be better and what would constitute success. Having a clear and agreed view of how we plan to improve services is vital. We also need to know what criteria we are going to use in order to make a judgement about the relative success or failure (worthwhileness) of our actions. Some criteria can and should be pre-specified. Other criteria might emerge naturally during the course of action.

2 *What practical action can we take that might lead to success?* This is about being realistic and pragmatic. Teams should be open to considering evidence from other team efforts, in order to learn more about what might work for them. Staff should ask themselves: 'What have other people done that we could try?' Confident and committed teams gather as many ideas as they can before they act. They also discuss their 'sphere of influence'. In other words, a team might usefully ask:

'What is it we feel we can do ourselves and what are the things we feel we need help with?'

3   *How will we know that something is a success?* This can be a tricky question. Clearly not all change is a success. Not all change improves the existing situation. Much depends on the evidence used to make such judgements and how it is interpreted. We must not forget that important attributes of either success or (relative) failure cannot always be easily measured.

The nature of the debates around the question 'Does reflection make a difference?' have changed radically in recent years. More specifically, debates about the nature of evidence, its use in healthcare and the call for evidence-based practice (Exworthy & Scott 2004) have served to focus minds and actions. Expectations are now high that any claims that reflection is good, useful, essential for learning and therefore justifiable, must be grounded in evidence. For some, these claims also have to be theoretically informed. The importance of reflective practices can no longer simply be juxtaposed with notions of staff-centredness, bottom-up and empowerment processes. Neither is reflection some kind of alternative to top-down, management-led modernisation. Modern forms of reflective practices blur this separation in a number of important ways, for example by becoming more inclusively participatory and by a broadening of its agenda to include issues of organisational governance, thereby linking with improvements in policy as well as practice. In turn, these shifts in attention invite us to engage with wider debates concerning the changing state and with UK Department of Health processes of democratisation and decentralisation (Department of Health 2004a, 2004b, 2004c, 2004d, 2004e, 2005). Bevington *et al.* (2004, p. 29) state that, 'In order to produce more rounded judgements on the performance of trusts, the NHS should work towards creating a collage of hard and soft data. Soft information is here to stay. The key to success is the degree of rigour and imagination involved in its collection, interpretation and use'.

Oldham (2004) offers a PDSA cycle to help achieve success. This is a traditional learning cycle where you 'Plan' a change, 'Do' it, 'Study' the results you get, and then 'Act' on the results. He emphasises small-scale improvement efforts and using many consecutive cycles to build up information about how effective the change is. He suggests that success is more likely to happen if we plan well, take small steps and use the PDSA cycle repeatedly. Oldham says this makes it easier to reduce the risk of something going wrong. What is overtly missing from each stage of the cycle is the necessity for collegial, team-based reflective learning conversations. These act as a comfort, give us courage to keep going or change the course of action in a principled manner and can be used to check that what we set out to do, is what we are still doing!

On learning through

Finally, this is a book informed by three mutually supportive 'learning through' processes. The key process is learning through the interests and practices of reflection (Part Two). Another concerns learning through working together in teams that are always developing in one way or another (Part Three). The third is about learning through an approach to better team learning based on the idea of 'wellness' and the 'healthy team'. This approach forms part of a facilitated, reflective process called **TA²LK** (IRP-UK 2005). **TA²LK** facilitates the development of reflective healthcare teams that are able to sustain high quality, personalised care (Part Four). It addresses this complex challenge in a flexible way.

Reflection is a catalyst for learning and a response to learning. It is also a matter of invention. By this I mean there are many ways to 'do' reflection. Much depends upon who is involved and why. The challenge is to develop the 'right' reflective processes, with the right people, at the right time and with the right purpose(s) in mind. This is a very value-laden enterprise. Additionally, the practices of team reflection may be considered as moral, ethical and intellectual. Therefore, specific conditions, or workplace cultures, are required for participation in them and to get the most from them. These conditions are not simply practical things like time and places to undertake reflection. Developing reflective teams also requires habits of mind, moral and intellectual dispositions and improving existing patterns of relationships. In many healthcare organisations efforts to establish and sustain cultures of reflection collide with hostile cultures of positivism, performance targets and means-ends instrumentalism. Those who advocate learning through the practices of reflection have to react, and respond positively and creatively, to such influences.

References

Barnett, R. (1996) *The Limits of Competence: Knowledge, Higher Education and Society*. The Society for Research into Higher Education & The Open University, Buckingham.

Bevington, J., Stanton, P. & Cullen, R. (2004) Gently does it. *Health Service Journal* 11 November.

Department of Health (2004a) *Better Information, Better Choices, Better Health: Putting Information at the Centre of Health*. DoH, London.

Department of Health (2004b) *Delivering HR in the NHS Plan: More Staff Working Differently*. DoH, London.

Department of Health (2004c) *Improving Hospital Doctor's Working Lives*. DoH, London.

Department of Health (2004d) *Putting People at the Heart of Public Services*. DoH, London.

Department of Health (2004e) *The NHS Improvement Plan: Putting People at the Heart of Public Services*. DoH, London.

Department of Health (2005) *Treatment Centres: Developing Faster, Quality Care and Choice for NHS Patients.* DoH, London.

Dewey, J. (1933) *How We Think: A Restatement of the Relation of Reflective Thinking to the Educative Process.* Heath & Company, Lexington, Massachesetts.

Exworthy, M. & Scott, T. (2004) The human touch. *Health Service Journal* 4 November.

IRP-UK (2005) *TA^{2}LK: The Essence of Improvement.* The Institute of Reflective Practice, IRP-UK Publications, Gloucester.

Nicolini, D., Sher, M., Childerstone, S. & Gorli, M. (2004) In search of the 'structure that reflects': promoting organizational reflection practices in a UK health authority. In *Organizing Reflection* (eds M. Reynolds & R. Vince). Ashgate Aldershot.

Oldham, J. (2004) Something to shout about. *Health Service Journal* 14 October: 20.

Reynolds, M. & Vince, R. (eds) (2004) *Organizing Reflection.* Ashgate Publishing, Aldershot.

Rosenfeld, J. & Tardieu, B. (2000) *Artisans of Democracy.* University Press of America, New York.

Schein, E. (1992) *Organisational Culture and Leadership.* Jossey-Bass, San Francisco.

Sitkin, S. (1996) Learning through failure: the strategy of small losses. In *Organisational Learning* (eds M. Cohen & L. Sproull). Sage, Thousand Oaks, California.

Chapter 2

Starting points:
through the learning lens

In this section I want to describe some of the book's general starting points. These are important because it looks at the development of reflective teams through some new and different lenses. The first is a *learning lens* because this is essentially a book about learning. Fig. 2.1 shows that there are three important constituents to this lens. The second is a *reflective lens*, where I begin to set out some ideas and processes that are explored in more depth in Part Two. The third is a *team lens*. I look at this in detail in Part Three.

(Re)focusing on learning

One thing we have in common is that we are all different. We see the world differently and do different things. For any one of the things we do, some of us do it better, others do it less well. It therefore follows that we may have learned to do it differently – some better, some worse. More precisely perhaps we have learned differently – some better, some worse. Learning is an experience. Reflective practices take experiences and help turn them into a special kind of learning. That is learning that we can make use of. Marton & Booth (1997) argue that there are different ways that we experience learning, for example through committing words, meanings and procedures to memory and then being able to reproduce them, in the right way, when needed. Another is the experience of gaining understanding and then being able to do something differently and do different things when called upon to do so. In the context of this book three of their key questions are highly relevant. They are;

1   How do we acquire what we learn?
2   In what forms does this learning persist?
3   How do we make use of this learning?

This book takes as a starting point, an holistic view of learning. In other words a view that all learning involves feeling, thinking and doing, although one aspect may be more dominant at any particular time. It also adopts a starting position that learning through reflective practices is dependent on perspective and experience and that it is an active and interactive process. Demarest *et al.* (2004) remind us that we cannot be of

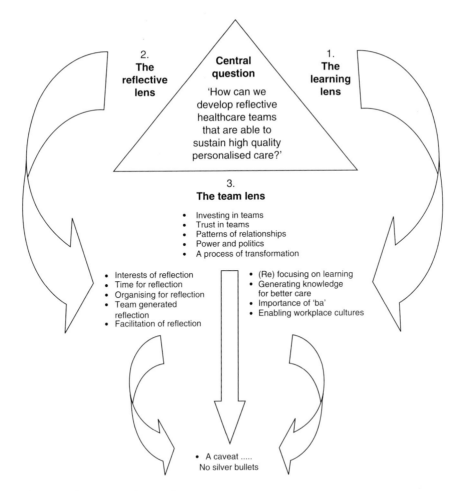

Fig 2.1 Some starting points.

much help to others, or ourselves, unless we are willing to be a learner at every moment. They offer us two challenges when they say that we need to recognise when we are 'lost' (when we don't know, when we get stuck and so on) and be open to learning from others. These are fundamental learning principles and central starting points for a book like this. They say we should, 'Be willing to be lost, to acknowledge that you don't know when you don't know, to approach relationships as an unfolding adventure and to listen to learn' (Demarest *et al.* 2004, p. vi). In many ways these challenges capture much of the essence of this book.

In the report of an expert group on learning from adverse events in the National Health Service in the UK (DoH 2000), there is an elaboration of the extent to which the health service has the ability to learn from such events. Failure to learn and the devastating consequences that arise from such failures are described as 'huge'. In the Executive Summary we find, 'Most distressing of all, such failures often have a familiar ring, displaying strong similarities to incidents which have occurred before and in some cases almost exactly replicating them. Many could be avoided if only the lessons of experience were properly learned' (DoH 2000, p. 1). Without investment in building sustainable cultures of team learning, it is hard to know how the Chief Medical Officer's report will be any different 10 years from now! A helpful distinction is made in this report (DoH 2000), between passive and active learning in the health service. The former is where lessons are identified but not put into practice. The latter is where those lessons are embedded into the organisation's culture and practices. So what gets in the way of more active learning? Better reporting systems are only one part of this. More fundamentally the root causes lie in the nature of organisational cultures. In this book I put forward the case that 'blame cultures' need to be transformed into cultures for reflective team learning. Understanding and transforming workplace cultures is an important feature of Part Four of this book. We should not forget that the cultures in the workplace are the most pervasive influence on how we feel and think and therefore on the quality of our actions there.

In the UKs Department of Health (2004b) publication called *Delivering HR in the NHS Plan: More Staff Working Differently*, there is a description of how the NHS aspires to become an employer of choice, a model employer and one that offers a model career to its staff. It proposes a strategy on how to achieve such a vision. It lays out the significant contribution that human resource management can make to patient care, brings a number of important workforce initiatives together and explicitly links the benefits to be had by staff and patients. At the heart of this strategy to modernise the health service in this way, we find the mantra of 'more staff, working differently'. Peeling this back reveals a commitment by government not only to its workforce but to creating new working environments. The purpose of this plan is to ensure effective, high quality personalised care. More staff alone will not modernise the health service. The key to success, the Department says, is in learning how to work differently. They argue that this does not simply mean the creation of new roles, but also the redesign of existing jobs to fit the skills and needs of staff more closely.

Currently, there are many initiatives designed to enable staff to work differently in the NHS. Agenda for Change, the Changing Workforce Programme, the Consultant Contract and Incentives Implementation, Protocol-Based Care, recruitment, retention and returning to work, and solutions to the European Working Time Directive are some of these initiatives (DoH 2004b). What binds all these initiatives together is a commitment to improving patient care. What will help or hinder the achievement of this commitment are at least three things. First are the opportunities staff have to learn together. Second is the quality of learning needed and wanted by staff. The need is clearly there (DoH 2001a).

For example, 1600 hospital doctors, in 2004, were asked what they wanted in a survey as part of the DoH-funded intercollegiate Improving Working Lives initiative (DoH 2004c). Education and training were thought to most improve the working lives of consultants, specialist registrars, senior house officers and pre-registration house officers and staff grade and associated specialities. This need is replicated elsewhere across the NHS. Third is leadership for and a collective commitment to improved action.

In analysing data for this book, I have come to believe that there are certain prerequisites for meaningful (team) learning. In other words the kind of learning that makes a real difference to care. Merely asking, supporting and encouraging staff to work differently (not just harder) is not enough. There appear to be particular aspects of task and team working (Groesbeck & van Aken 2001), supported by a core of agreed values, for this to be a success. I explore these in some detail in Parts Three and Four when I discuss the development of reflective healthcare teams in relation to the idea of values team wellness.

Generating knowledge for better care

Another important starting point is the basic view that the practices of reflection involve learning from reflections on what we do. This is not as straightforward as it seems (see Part Two). As I mentioned earlier these practices cannot be characterised merely as focusing on problems to be solved. They are far more involving than simply thinking in this way about our work and obsessions with the 'quick fix'. To be useful in the demanding world of healthcare, reflection needs to be something other than just 'thinking about practice'. Crucially it is also about the way practices of reflection enable us to generate actionable knowledge to improve services and workplaces in particular experiential contexts. A further starting point then is to see this knowledge as something that is created or made, not just collected. In this book I take a position that knowledge is created by teams (and groups) of people who share a language and a perspective (Slife & Williams 1995). This is a social constructionist position (Velody & Williams 1998). Allied to this is a view of knowledge as constantly open to revision and to interpretation. This way of knowing does not occur within individuals. It occurs in the relationships among individuals as they converse, negotiate, practise their skills and share views of their worlds with one another. It follows that the 'knowing' in reflective teams might usefully be understood in terms of socially constructed, team-relative knowledge. One consequence of this is that the knowledge that teams create may well contradict earlier and much cherished knowledge that guides and informs their practice. Additionally, Parker (1997) reminds us that within what we take to be a single practice, there can be multiple and incompatible realities.

There are of course many ways of knowing and we should not celebrate any of them uncritically. As with every way of knowing, there are limitations to them. The same can be said of a constructionist position. For example, Morss (1996, p. 45) states, 'The term "social construction" has begun to sound a little tired, and its repetition threatens to turn it into dogma. There is a kind of stubborn humanism and an optimism that is sometimes a little cloying. There is a tendency to self-centredness that sometimes prevents a scrutiny of the positioning of self within larger structures of society'. A problem with a constructionist view is that it suggests that people are free to negotiate social reality between themselves. Also there is an assumption that people interact on equal terms. 'Pretending that people are equal goes alongwith pretending that they can control their own lives. The social constructionists make out that people are voluntary, rational agents, choosing freely among a range of alternatives.... If people could control their own lives, how many would choose the lives they have?' (Morss 1996, p. 55).

A social constructionist view also has to deal with the important issue of relativism. By this I mean that it is one thing to acknowledge that social reality and knowledge are constructed. It is quite another to say that these constructions are true, right, good or useful. So there may be little or no justification for claiming that one specific theory or view of knowledge is a better representation of 'reality' than another. Hence we may have to reject scientific claims to 'objective truth'. The work of Foucault (1977) and Rainbow (1991) are particularly useful in helping us understand this issue. They both suggest that our personal and collective identities and practices reflect conflicts and tensions between the 'dominated' and the 'dominating'. These issues are particularly relevant when developing healthcare teams.

A further issue is that, for some, the generation of knowledge is not about the search for the truth (on the matter) but simply a process to try to get the upper hand on, and the high ground over, other teams. Here knowledge becomes part of a more general struggle between teams for notoriety, for securing increasingly scarce resources, for exclusivity and elitism. When this is the case we often find team members speaking to each other, and about practice, in coded familiarity. Unlike some other ways of knowing like empiricism (which appeals to common experience) or rationality (which appeals to common sense), a social constructionist view appeals most often to pragmatism. In other words what seems ton work most effectively, efficiently and successfully for us within particular settings and workplace cultures. This pragmatism also includes issues to do with what works in the best interests of patients, clients, carers, families and so on. Whatever knowledge we use, it must be open to challenge and reconstruction. This means that values, traditions, understandings, identities and actions all have to be continuously reviewed. Durability of ideas and practices is no criterion of worth.

It is also well known that learners actively construct and deconstruct their experience (Taylor 1997). The major influence on learning is the learner's 'personal foundation of experience' (Boud & Walker 1990) and the cumulative effect this has on how we feel and think and therefore what we can do in certain healthcare contexts. Two particular points made by Boud *et al.* (1993) and Taylor (1997) are highly relevant to the process of developing reflective teams. First is the influence of past experience, which sets expectations for the present and future about what can and cannot be achieved. Second, there is the influence of the current context, which mediates the effect of past experience and may either support or inhibit the way staff move forward.

The importance of 'ba' (a place, context or setting)

Von Krogh *et al.* (2000) draw upon the Japanese idea of 'ba' when making the point that effective knowledge creation depends upon the nature of particular contexts. For healthcare teams, 'ba' is a shared knowledge generating space. They go on to suggest that managers need to support knowledge creation rather than try to control it. They call this process 'knowledge enabling'. They identify five kinds of knowledge enablers. These are (i) instil a knowledge vision, (ii) manage conversations, (iii) mobilise knowledge activists, (iv) create the right context, and (v) globalise local knowledge. However, the key to all this happening is the development of a kind of emotional literacy (see Part Four) that highlights how staff treat each other. They argue that knowledge creation has to happen in a caring context. In Part Four I describe five attributes necessary for teams to become more emotionally literate. Collectively I place them in what I call the team's 'care zone'. Good health in the care zone provides a basis for thinking and acting differently. This, in turn, helps teams make a difference to practice and policy.

So a further starting point for this book is a reaffirmation of the importance of context. As I mentioned earlier, I take a view that all learning is socially and culturally constructed *in a context*. In this book I also view healthcare contexts as essentially dynamic, where individual and collective values and actions serve to give it a unity and where patterns of interaction can reveal internal disunity and diversity (see Part Four). Turning experience into learning is inevitably therefore influenced by context. This might be an historical-cultural context, a socio-emotional context, a workplace practice, a policy imperative, target driven, financially constrained context and so on. This is particularly crucial to understand in healthcare as practitioners work with patients, clients, carers, families and colleagues who have values (and therefore actions) shaped by their personally experienced context or situation. Understanding the influence of context may directly influence a specific judgement made, or a course of action taken. Reflective practices always take place in a context. In healthcare these are extremely varied.

Enabling workplace cultures

A further starting point is to ask the general question: 'What is the proper focus for improving services?' In this book I set the development of reflective teams, not in what some regard as the politically correct context of organisational structures but in an increasingly significant and tangible cultural context. This again poses a number of structure-culture dilemmas for us. Plsek *et al*. (2004) argue that an emphasis on structure can underestimate the power of existing patterns of working and learning that profoundly shape current practice. Consequently they can over-estimate the power of structural change to alter such practice. This situation generates a troublesome image of a powerful, determining structure acting on a relatively malleable body of practice. In this scenario the key to change is getting the structure(s) right so they support the organisation's goals (or mission), then have practice conform to them. There is nothing inherently good or bad about focusing on structures and re-structuring. Much depends on who controls them, who is participating in them and the purposes to which structures are put. We can have re-structuring as a form of bureaucratic control with staff and service users being (c)overtly controlled and regulated. Alternatively we can develop structures for empowerment that support staff and users by creating opportunities for dialogue and for making improvements to practice and policy. A focus on transforming workplace cultures is not dilemma-free either. Just like a focus on re-structuring, it brings with it dilemmas that involve ethics and political choices about values and purposes. There is also a basic duality about organisational cultures. On the one hand they make complex interactions and coordination of health-care services possible. On the other hand they can be constraining and repressive.

A recently concluded study by Joyce *et al*. (2003) called *The Evergreen Project* links culture with structure in an important way. Generally their findings have implications for those striving to sustain high, health service performance. They ask the question: What really works for sustained business success? They focused on success (see Chapter 1) and what really worked for 160 companies over a 10-year period. They found there were four basic archetypes: winners, climbers, tumblers and losers. Data from surveys, in-depth studies of management practices and document analyses enabled them to came up with their 4 + 2 Formula. They found eight management practices, four primary (culture, structure, strategy and execution) and four secondary practices (talent management, leadership, innovation and mergers and partnerships) that directly correlated with superior corporate performance. All four primary practices are a must for success and any two of the four secondary practices. Hence their 4 + 2 formula. With regard to the importance of culture they recommend:

- Inspire all managers and employees to do their best.
- Empower staff and managers to make independent decisions and to find ways to improve practices, including their own.
- Reward achievement with pay based on performance, but keep raising the performance bar.
- Pay psychological rewards in additional to financial ones.
- Create a challenging, satisfying work environment.
- Establish and abide by clear company values.

In Parts Three and Four of this book I will explore how some of these primary and secondary practices are of relevance to the development of reflective teams. At this point it is worth stressing two things. Developing high-performing reflective teams is not simply about what members choose to do. It is also about how well they sustain these practices (Bevington 2005).

Organisational cultures affect the quality of care. So understanding their creation and maintenance matters. 'A cultural change is not that management tries to impose new behaviours, but a change of the ideas, values and meanings of large groups of people' (Alvesson 2003, p. 173). We should also note that creating cultures that enable staff to maximise their contributions to care is a major, long-term challenge in itself. Cultures take time to change. Open, fair and blame-free cultures are much talked about within the NHS. They cannot be created overnight. But what are their attributes? (See Part Four.) Working differently (DoH 2004b) suggests that the government welcomes and needs to encourage a plurality of cultures, eroding the once pervasive command-and-control one. The implication is that spaces will need to be created to discuss things like whose interests are being served, conflict between staff groups, things like privilege, exploitation, oppression and domination within and between professions. Creating more enabling cultures is fundamentally about making the axes of power transparent within and between particular disciplines and healthcare organisations. This requires working hard to understand how knowledge, power and experience affect staff and user empowerment and service improvement in everyday practice settings.

What seems to be at stake here, behind the rhetoric of working differently, is not the mere recognition of difference. Nor is it simply that staff in more enabling cultures have a voice. I suggest the more crucial question concerns the sort of voice we come to have as a result of being part of such cultures, both as individuals and as members of a team. At the very least this needs to be an active, sometimes oppositional and collective voice. By oppositional I do not mean either constantly contesting mainstream (or *male*stream) thinking and practice. Nor do I mean being radical and subversive in a kind of avant-garde sense of 'shocking', vis-à-vis conventional ways of doing things. I mean teams that stay attuned to the best of what the mainstream has to offer, its customs and practices, and teams that cultivate critical and creative sensibilities and collective accountability that encourages idea generation, curiosities and individual expressions. What the data for this book suggest is that enabling cultures are indeed enabling because they infuse staff (and significant others) with the self-confidence and capacity necessary for success without an undue reliance on the mainstream for approval and acceptance. They are cultures that need and nurture reflection. There is a symbiotic relationship between such cultures and reflective teams with one informing, transforming and sustaining the other.

We must not forget that the reproduction and maintenance of some workplace cultures is also an important task. Cultural maintenance means doing something positive when we feel we are drifting away from core values and agreed practices. Maintenance is required when shared meanings and ways of working get blurred and differentiated, making confusion and conflict more prevalent. So all this talk about culture change within the National Health Service needs to be balanced with processes for cultural maintenance. These include:

- Upholding particular values and maintaining morale in order to help staff do the best they can.
- Maintaining a team's identity in a complex and changing healthcare organisation and in so doing, enabling staff to hang on to the essence of what the team stands for and does.
- Sustaining the team's image or 'profile' in relation to the work of other teams and groups of staff.

Chapter 3
Through the reflective lens

Clarifying some interests in the practices of reflection

Reflection has a longer genealogy in thinking and practice than is usually acknowledged. This is an important recognition because much of the focus on reflection and reflective practices during the 1990s tended to emphasise three things: self–reflection, personal reflective writing and critiques of it (Bleakley 2000, Johns 2000, 2002, Landes & English 2000, Stapleton-Watson & Wilcox 2000, Taylor 2000, Bolton 2001, Burns & Bulman 2001, Kember *et al.* 2001, McCormack 2001, Stuart 2001, Glaze 2002, Loo & Thorpe 2002, Longnecker 2002, Risner 2002, Tsang 2003, Krmpotić-Schwind 2003, Shepherd 2004, Moon 2004, Gully 2004, Thorpe 2004). These emphases still persist. One consequence of this has been that some have regarded these practices as sufficient and as a definitive form of reflection. In this book I support those practices of reflection that enable teams to make improvements in services and workplaces. By necessity then the view is fairly catholic. Parker (1997) begins to capture some of the essentials of this when he talks about practices that have a commitment to the authority of reason, which favour a concern with ends and values, which reject a technical-rationalist view of human worth and enable us to exercise both autonomy and responsibility. I discuss these in more detail in Part Two. All I want to do here is signal some of the influences that have had an impact on some current interests of reflective practices and particularly those for service and workplace improvement. Briefly stated the following are pertinent.

Technical rationality

This is still pervasive in healthcare. In general it embraces the philosophy of positivism. What this means is that the procedures we use and the quality standards we employ are those of the natural sciences. It is also based on a conception of rationality as a process of working out the most efficient means of achieving pre-specified and thereby knowable ends. It takes ends as given and outside the scope of rational scrutiny. The power of rationality is judged '. . . solely in terms of the efficiency of means in achieving ends' (Siegel 1988, p. 130). Derived from this is a view of a healthcare professional as a means-end broker, with healthcare as a technical 'delivery system'. Donald Schön rejected technical rationalism and its value-free notion of efficiency and effectiveness.

Realism

This is linked with positivism and the practices of technical rationalism. Realism has a central belief that the world exists around us and 'out there', independently of our mind, social and healthcare practices and our lives. It is, '... indifferent to whatever we happen to believe about it at any particular moment... The world exists independently of the perceptions, actions and statements of this or that group, culture or individual... [it is an]... independent yardstick against which we must measure our beliefs in establishing their truth and falsity... Thus we make discoveries about it' (Parker 1997, p. 21). Realism is still pervasive in much of healthcare.

Intentional pursuit

John Dewey (1916) described learning as the '... intentional pursuit of a course of action' (p. 138), an example of an intentional pursuit being improving services and workplaces. Dewey saw such a pursuit as a relationship between trying things out and then reflecting on the consequences, not in a haphazard and arbitrary manner, but a systematic, step-by-step one. This is the emergence of what some call action-as-research (Winter & Munn-Giddings 2001). Dewey describes reflection on intentional action as involving a '... sense of problem, the observation of conditions, the formation and rational elaboration of a suggested conclusion' (Dewey 1916, p. 151). Much of this thinking evidences itself today in the work of action researchers (Ghaye & Wakefield 1993, Whitehead 1993, Zuber-Skerritt 1996 Reason & Bradbury 2001, Day *et al.* 2002). Dewey was opposed to the idea of 'routine action', which he saw as being dominated by '... tradition, habit and authority and by institutional definitions and expectations' (Pollard & Tann 1994, p. 9). He put forward a view that practising reflection required three particular personal qualities. These are:

1 *Open-mindedness*, which enables us to be receptive to different views on significant issues. It is an openness to a plurality of ways of noticing, understanding and working towards improving services.
2 *Responsibility* in pursuing intentional action designed to bring about improvements in practice. This involves putting our achievements and successes 'under pressure' from public scrutiny.
3 *Wholeheartedness* in our commitment to pursue something worthwhile.

The critical being

Critical reflection is gaining popularity. It is caught up with terms like emancipation and liberation. The theoretical underpinning for it is offered by critical theory. This involves a look at the way history, identity construction, power, politics and different discourses for example, affect the way we feel, think and act in particular settings. Relatively recently the practices of reflection have been informed by the critical being movement (Carr & Kemmis 1986, Fay 1987, Ghaye 1995, Brookfield 1995, 2000a, 2000b, Ghaye & Ghaye 1998, Rolfe et al. 2001). There are different versions of this movement in different disciplines, but Barnett (1997) suggests that there are three fundamental parts of the critical being. They are critical thought, critical (self)reflection and critical action. Put another way, these are about particular kinds of self and collective thinking and action.

So what might critical reflection be? Rolfe *et al.* (2001, p. xi) hold Barnett's three ideas together when they define it as '... using the reflective process to look systematically and rigorously at our own practice'. They go on to say that, 'We all reflect on our practice to some extent, but how often do we employ those reflections to learn from our actions, to challenge established theory and, most importantly, to make a real difference to our practice?'. The ways of looking they outline are suggestive of a critical frame of mind, a general critical disposition. Barnett (1997, p. 87) describes this as '... an ability to size up the world in its different manifestations and the capacity to respond in different ways... the willingness to evaluate the world, howsoever it appears'. For me this critical disposition also includes our ability to critique a body of knowledge and routine customs and practice. Some important related questions are:

- What is involved in critical consciousness? (Johns & Freshwater 1998).
- How can we avoid a situation of being reflective but thoroughly uncritical? (Barnett 1997).
- How can we remain critical and yet optimistic? (Brookfield 2000b).

Later in this book I will talk in more detail about the work of Paulo Freire (1972, 1974, 1994, 1998, Freire & Macedo 1998) and the way his ideas of emancipation and critical consciousness are relevant to the development of reflective healthcare teams. For now it is worth mentioning that there are some powerful legacies of the critical being from Freire. His emphasis on meaningful dialogue, on the process of problematization and questioning the world, are highly relevant to improving healthcare today. A critical disposition helps to make us more aware that our practices could be other than they are. This disposition usually draws in big ideas like power, empowerment and ideology. These help us understand that the current state of play, in particular healthcare settings, is the result of historical and uneven forces. 'This ability to become critically conscious is far removed from simply examining an event to see what should be done differently. There is an implicit political dimension, linked to critical awareness, which enables assumptions inherent in ideologies to be challenged' (Johns & Freshwater 1998, p. 152).

This kind of challenge means action must be critical action. But can action in the National Health Service be of this kind? Critical action is linked to a team's capacity to see themselves in new ways and to do different things. Arguably critical action is about engaging in '... *disruptive, sceptical and "other" social and discourse relations than those dominant, conventionalised and extant in particular fields...*' (Luke 2004 p. 26). In doing so we need to be mindful of Brookfield's (2000b, p. 145) point that this might be energy-sapping with staff leaving themselves '... *feeling puny, alone, vulnerable and demoralised in the face of structural power that seems overwhelming and unchangeable*'. For critical action to happen we need to find ways to step outside the frame of 'normal practices' and put on reflective lenses that help make the familiar and conventional strange. This 'strangeness' might help us ask serious questions about practice, what it is like and how it has come to be the way it is. Critical action can be risky if done alone. It can quickly lead to stress and burnout. For staff who feel oppressed, marginalised and silenced, this might be a real way to try to collectively move forward. So some of the important elements of critical action, which we need to carry forward in this book are that it is about:

- the political and trying to lobby for and influence change;
- constantly holding under review (critiquing) our relationship with service structures and systems; and
- engaging positively with forms of political oppression and repression in the places where we work and particularly in debates about who gets what, where and how.

Empowerment

Empowerment is a complex idea and interacts with the previous notion of the critical being and the following process of being creative. In the context of developing healthcare teams we need to ask two fundamental questions: Who feels empowered and why? Talk of empowerment has been fashionable for some time. Throughout much of the literature on empowerment there is an assumption that it is a 'good thing'. Some argue that it is better to be empowered than disempowered. But do staff and service users want to feel more empowered? What assumptions are we making here? One senior clinician said to me recently, 'All this talk of empowering my staff. What's going to happen if they then turn round and start asking me questions I can't answer?' Some say that being empowered is about being more effective, productive, fulfilled and healthier. This broad conception of empowerment has been described as a 'myopia of therapeutic good intention' (Jack 1995). When associated with the individual, empowerment is often called 'self-empowerment'. This term is linked to ideas of self-care, self-responsibility, self-determination, and personal control and struggle (Kendall 1998). It is to do with individuals taking control of their circumstances, achieving their personal desires and goals and trying to enhance the quality of their lives (Adams 1990). But this book goes beyond individualism. Team empowerment is often experienced in terms of the quality of relationships between staff and what these enable them to do in their practice. This is also linked with the idea of an empowering partnership (Tones 1993, Le May 1998), which may occur, for example, in certain nurse/patient relationships, between trusts and across health economies.

One enduring problem with empowerment is that it is often seen as a commodity, bestowed on those without it, by those who have it to give. It is a commodity that is given or withheld. If you have it, you are empowered. If not, then you are disempowered. This is a crude and simplistic view, linked to the consumer movement in healthcare in the 1980s and 90s. If empowerment is seen as something bestowed on healthcare staff and their patients/clients by those people who have it to give, rather than as something personally acquired through struggle and negotiation, then it might be better to regard it as just another form of social control or oppression (Ghaye & Ghaye 1998, Piper & Brown 1998). It might be more helpful to regard empowerment as a process where, for instance, staff teams transform themselves in some beneficial manner. This usually involves some commitment to a 'cause', a group of patients/clients, or to a vision. The actual process can involve certain strategies or steps. These again can be problematic. For example, some describe this as a 'pass-it-on' process. This finds expression thus: 'Nurses themselves must first be empowered in order to be able to empower others' (Latter 1998, p. 24). Another example is the 'give-it-away' process. Again, this finds expression in such phrases as, 'We have to relinquish power, our role as expert, and pass control over to others'. This, of course, is potentially threatening for both parties.

We can also find evidence of empowerment described as an 'enablement' process. This view asserts that the process is not so much about giving power away, as about creating opportunities that enable and encourage power to be taken. Then there is empowerment as 'a process of becoming' (Keiffer 1984). Keiffer describes the empowerment process as having four stages. First, there is an exploratory stage where authority and power structures are demystified. It is a kind of reconnaissance stage. Second, there is an 'era of advancement', where strategies for action are developed. Third comes an 'era of incorporation' in which the barriers to increased self-determination are confronted. Finally, we have an 'era of commitment', where new knowledge and skills help to create new realities. In an interesting book by Johnson and Redmond (1998), empowerment is described as an 'art' and the pinnacle of staff involvement. They argue that the process whereby an organisation moves away from a hierarchical 'command and control' culture towards one of empowerment, is associated with employee 'profit and pain' and a shift in the existing power matrix. Empowering staff often involves a change in management style. It certainly involves a change in the cultures within organisations.

In this book I offer the following view of empowerment. Empowerment is about teams coming to know, expressing and critically analysing their own realities and having the commitment, will and power to act to transform these realities, to enhance personal and collective well-being, security, satisfaction, capability and working conditions. Naturally this view raises such questions as: Whose reality? Whose reality counts? Discussions about empowerment inevitably involve notions of power: what it is, who has and does not have it, who wants it and cannot get it, who has it and does not want it and who does what with it. Power is a complex and slippery notion. For some it is about sectional interests, territoriality, giving and gaining ground, about domination and dependence. When these are understood in relation to team empowerment, it takes us into the hugely important area of social justice (Griffiths 1998). In essence, enhancing social justice through becoming more empowered, means that team members have to understand and alter some of the existing patterns of power relations.

One characteristic of members of reflective teams is that they think about ways to constructively resist, confront and alter those patterns that serve to constrain thinking and action in certain healthcare settings. So empowerment is associated with voice. Voice can be regarded as the connection between reflection and action. If team members feel that they are staff upon whom power is brought to bear to ensure their compliance and 'domesticity' to prevailing values and routines, then their voice is as one of the oppressed (Ryles 1999). Challenging this hegemony is about developing a voice and making it heard. 'This, it can be argued, will be achieved by a commitment to the raising of political consciousness within nurses as a means of not only having them recognise the current nature of their position but also beginning to challenge and change those circumstances' (Ryles 1999, pp. 605–606). In this sense, 'voice' is used to enable team members to resist becoming colonised or domesticated by an elite and put in the service of maintaining their interests and perhaps the status quo.

By implication then, empowerment is not simply a process of 'giving a voice'; it is more complicated than this. Habermas (1977) argued that power is often exercised through the manipulation and/or distortion of patterns of communication. In reality this can mean the power to control agendas, to use personal knowledge possessed by the privileged few, through authority. This connects with Luke's (1974) view about the way powerful elite groups are able to persuade less powerful groups to hold views or act in ways that are contrary to their own interests. In the context of the UK government's commitment to modernize the health service, it is critical that we strive to understand whose interests are being served and what patterns of power, communication and decision-making underlie this.

Creativity

The practices of reflection should not just be critical. They must also be creative. The need for continuous improvements in practice and policy leads directly to the need for ideas for improvement. But generating ideas requires effort and a productive process. A problem is that while many staff have the ability to think in new ways, see things differently and to imagine better ways of practising, they are often locked into existing patterns of thinking. This may be due to habit. It takes an effort to break out of this. It may be that in their workplace the knowledge enabling processes (see earlier) are poor. So it is in no way helpful to simply urge staff to 'think outside the box'. When we need a creative idea, it does little good to tell ourselves, and others, to just think harder. We have to think differently. Part of the trick is to be alive to opportunities to be creative. Drucker (1985) calls these 'innovative opportunities'. Some opportunities like this can come from within the team. For example they may:

1 *Be unexpected.* Arising from unforeseen success or failure, a new member's contribution to the team and so on.
2 *Arise from incongruence.* A puzzling or worrying gap between what staff say and do, what is and what ought to be.
3 *Stem from a practice need.* Something a team does routinely becomes inefficient or ineffective and needs to change.
4 *Be generated through the practices of reflection.* From reflections on the way the team puts its values into action.

Other innovative opportunities can originate from outside the team. For example they may:

5 *Be policy driven.* From a decision to implement a local or national policy imperative. For example, the local implementation of a single assessment process for older people as a response to the National Service Framework (DoH 2001b).
6 *Arise from demographic changes.* In the socio-economic status, mortality and ethnicity of people in the community and across the health economy.
7 *Be linked with greater public participation and changes in perception.* For example as associated with the establishment of The Commission for Patient and Public Involvement and the Patient and Public Involvement (PPI) Forums in every NHS Trust and Primary Care Trust (PCT) in England.
8 *Associated with the creation and dissemination of 'new' knowledge and procedures.* For example through the work of the National Institute for Clinical Excellence, the NHS Health Development Agency, the National Patient Safety Agency, the Improvement Partnership for Ambulance Services, the National Health Service University (NHSU)/NHS Modernisation Agency and the work of the Leadership Centre.

There are many knowledge enabling processes that help us to be more creative. For example, there is brainstorming, kinds of reframing matrix activities, concept fans, random input tasks and provocation techniques. The use of de Bono's Six Thinking Hats can be particularly helpful. For more details consult (http://www.edwdebono.com/) and (www.holst-group.co.uk). The use of his thinking hats is supportive of efforts to modernise healthcare and sustain improvements. The hats help us generate;

- more quality new ideas;
- more creative solutions;
- greater involvement from everyone;
- better quality decision-making; and
- less frustrating unproductive, adversarial debate.

The six thinking hats use parallel thinking as an alternative to (and not a replacement for) traditional ways of thinking. Parallel thinking is often more productive than adversarial thinking, argument or debate. There are six different coloured hats that can be put on or taken off as team members focus on something of concern that they wish to 'move forward'. Each hat represents a different type or mode of thinking. The whole team wears the same colour hat and changes hats at the same time.

New workplace cultures that enable us to be more creative may have to be simultaneously supportive and pushy, anxiety provoking and anxiety containing. But to think differently and act differently is inherently risky. This takes us back again to the idea I mentioned earlier about 'failure' (see Orientation). Martin (2003) takes this further when saying that failure is governed by four values:

1   To *win and not lose* in any interaction.
2   To always *maintain control* of the situation in hand.
3   To avoid *embarrassment* of any kind.
4   To *stay rational* throughout.

(Martin 2003, p. 34, italics in original)

Everyday we might have to decide whether to put our creative contributions 'out there', or keep them to ourselves to avoid upsetting anyone. In doing this we can (hopefully) get through another day. In many healthcare settings it is right to be cautious. Prudence is a virtue. We can disturb people when we bring provocative and new ideas to team meetings, when we question the gap between members' values and practices. We risk being marginalised and can make ourselves vulnerable when we do this.

So things are beginning to fit. The basic human tendency is to avoid and attempt to eliminate or ignore fear, a sense of vulnerability and anxiety. Arguably these are precisely what are not needed in situations of healthcare modernisation. Staff who are creative can be seen as 'rocking the boat'. They can 'get up your nose'. But these people are needed every bit as much as like-minded staff. Team leaders and senior managers, because they are in positions of authority and power should, I suggest, role model new governing values based on relational trust (Reina & Reina 1999), creativity and disciplined confrontation of problems and concerns. In Part Four I explore this in more detail when I describe three important constituents that appear to have a direct bearing on a team's capability to think differently. Collectively I place them in what I call the team's 'creative zone'. Good health in this zone helps teams make a difference to practice and policy.

Time for reflection

Developing reflective learning healthcare teams is, by its very nature, suggestive of a process that takes time. This process is commonly described in terms of linear, stage or life-cycle models (Kur 1996) with Tuckman's (1965, Tuckman & Jenson 1977) 'forming', 'storming', 'norming' and 'performing' being a classic example. His model describes teams as moving through a step-by-step, or sequential, one-way development pattern over time. Without doubt we need to appreciate that the temporal dynamics of team development are important because they help us understand how personal and collective histories, the demands of practice and unfolding policy imperatives, impact on developing more team-based work cultures. Time is needed to enable loose staff groups to become effective and reflective teams (Sheard & Kakabadse 2002). This does not happen overnight. Teams, yet alone reflective ones, cannot be created at a stroke; only groups can be formed in this way. The benefits of team working also take time to emerge. What complicates and undermines the development of teams is the way 'calendar time' is confused with 'practical time'. The pressing daily operational needs of clinical practice often force us into a mindset of time being linear and continuous. Calendar time is often imposed on practical or 'real' time. The latter is the time we really have to develop and sustain teams, to understand, negotiate and liberate the gifts and talents that staff have.

Organising for reflective practices

Reynolds and Vince (2004, p. 1) make the point that, '... *less emphasis needs to be placed on reflection as the task of individuals and more emphasis needs to be put on creating collective and organisationally focused processes for reflection. Another way of saying this is: less about the individual reflective practitioner and more about organizing reflection*'. In developing this idea they raise several helpful questions, namely:

- How far can reflection be a stable and self-sustaining process?
- To what extent is it possible to 'unsettle conventional practices' through organising reflection (and thereby promote organisational level learning)?

● How might individuals organise critical/collective reflection in order to challenge assumptions and to enrich approaches to education and development?

● How can organisational members better learn to challenge and be challenged? (Reynolds & Vince 2004, p. 11).

In general it is possible to think about engaging with reflective practices in at least eight ways, in terms of:

1 *The LOCUS of engagement.* For example, undertaken by an individual healthcare professional, or group, working in a particular setting. This, for example, places 'local' constructions of reality at the heart of the reflective process.

2 *The LEVEL of engagement.* For example, the department, unit, clinic, centre, hospital, community and so on. This raises the question: Who is, or should be, involved and what will be the focus of reflection? When considering the level of engagement we also have to consider issues of participation, empowerment, coercion and control.

3 *The MOTIVE(S) for engagement.* Why reflect? Why bother? Or do we just 'do it anyway?' Can reflection become more 'relevant' in terms of directly informing decision-making and enabling us to make wiser interventions? This motive of relevance is linked, in part, to a strong clinical imperative that reflective practices need to focus on solutions to new and on-going problems. But to privilege reflective practices in this way distracts attention from many of the other things in the worlds of working life that deserve our full attention, for example nurturing and sustaining our successes.

4 *The RIGHTS to engagement.* For example, the way teams struggle to find the time to come together to learn from reflection, the way it is added on to an already (over)crowded working life. The way the practices of reflection are seen as optional, done in staff's own time, discontinuous and therefore potentially disorganised. However, in policy statements like *Liberating the Talents* (DoH 2002b) and in initiatives like 'protected learning time' we find opportunities and arguments for reflection to be regarded as a basic professional 'right'.

5 *The RULES of engagement.* We should not demonize those with whom we disagree and should avoid affronting their deepest sensibilities. LePage & Sockett (2002) suggest that through the use of '*reconciliatory discourse*' (RD) we can make dialogue and conversation more constructive. At the heart of this is a commitment by participants (with divergent views) to seek to build a common ground to which they are morally and intellectually committed. There is a respect for diversity of views. They are treated positively (see Part Four). The overall purpose is to collectively make better judgements about practice. What I like about RD is that it goes beyond simply seeking common ground. The rules are to seek reconciliation on that common ground. Compromise, with its sense of a 'middle way', also is not enough. They argue that we

can compromise out of fear, not in a spirit of reconciliation. We can find '... common ground as a practical matter, but not take it seriously. Reconciliation, to repeat, demands a meeting of hearts as well as minds. It suggests commitment' (Le Page & Sockett 2002, p. 16). They go on to explain 'Reconciliation has its roots firmly planted in the idea that no matter what option we choose, we should be building on the morally and intellectually best in the different positions, such that we can each embrace the choices made' (Le Page & Sockett 2002, p. 19).

6 *The RESOURCES for engagement.* We need to avoid getting caught by talk of reflective tools and by images of mere behavioural accomplishments, of techniques to get by with. The practices of reflection are fundamentally about the kinds of healthcare professionals we are trying to educate and wish to see in practice.

7 *The IMPACT of engagement.* A new 'bottom line' for teams learning through the practices of reflection is to demonstrate real, worthwhile and sustainable differences to practice.

8 *The MORAL IMPERATIVE for engagement.* In addressing the central question of this book (see Fig. 2) there is a danger of teams losing their moral compass. One of the great strengths team members need to have, especially in times of healthcare modernisation, is a strong sense of moral purpose. This does not mean being saintly. It means keeping some fundamental questions in the forefront of our minds. Questions like: Why did I become a healthcare professional in the first place? What do I stand for as a team leader or manager? What legacy do I want to leave? (Livsey & Palmer 1999). The important point Block (2002) makes is that we too readily look to a how-to culture to obtain an answer, thereby suppressing deeper deliberations of intention, purpose and responsibility. In responding positively to the central question of this book, staff must not forget to ask the 'why' question. There are real dangers in getting lost in the 'how-to' questions. Talking about 'why' is using our moral compass well. It keeps us on a moral journey.

Team-generated reflection

Reflection may be done by oneself, alone or with others. This book emphasises the latter. It is a starting point that views the practice of reflection as an essentially public, team-based conversational enterprise. Unfortunately, much of the debate in the field of learning through reflection still tends to swing wildly between uncritical advocacy or outright rejection of reflection. In some academic and practitioner circles reflection is still dismissed as airy-fairy, subjective self-indulgence that can be very uncomfortable. For some it is synonymous with any old example of 'thinking again about what one is doing'. Some teachers of reflective practices are accused of dressing it up in a kind of mysterious psychobabble to try to give it an air of respectability. Also there are people who are very impatient with the process of reflecting on experience. They want the process to change their worlds, and now! Others may view it as an unwelcome diversion from the real and pressing needs of caring for patients because 'this is what I am paid to do'.

However, in other disciplines and workplaces reflection, of one kind or another, is as ubiquitous as ever. Recent developments in the general areas of lifelong learning, medical education, the work of the Health Professions Council in the UK and continuous professional development for example, have deepened and extended the role of reflection in learning. This has been accompanied by a range of new practices of reflection in a variety of settings such as the conventional 'classroom', in clinical areas and in the community. In general this book seeks to offer some alternatives to the critique ranged against reflection and more specifically against the reflective practitioner (reflection undertaken by individuals).

Schön's notion of the reflective practitioner (Schön 1998) has been a hugely constructive catalyst for thinking and action over the years. His work essentially concerned the exercise of human agency in relation to personal and professional development. In other words he recognised and celebrated the capacities and motivations of individuals, as active and intentional people, willing and perhaps able to understand themselves better and improve themselves and their work. Schön's views embody an optimistic vision of human potential. It is a view of individual practitioners who are, 'adaptive, but not passively, celebrating change and taking the initiative in its promotion' (Parker 1997, p. 6). Schön's work has been a particularly visible and mainstream variant of reflective practice in healthcare and is tied in closely with self-reflection. This has a double aspect. 'It calls forth a chosen action from the myriad of identified possibilities (now evaluated and discarded by the professional self) and it puts that choice into action' (Barnett 1997, p. 98). These two aspects of evaluation and execution can happen in the moment as with Schön's notion of reflection-in-action (see Part Two).

Whilst many of his original ideas and processes are still useful and appropriate, the worlds of healthcare delivery, management and development in the twenty-first century are now demanding new and different (some may argue complementary) approaches to learning through reflection. In addressing these concerns, the book seeks to establish reflection as a collegial and collective process. As Carini (2001) says, when we learn in the company of others we learn that each of us sees the world only partially, no matter how present we are to it. '*I learn that when I see a lot, I am still seeing only a little and partially. I learn that when others join in, the description is always fuller than what I saw alone*' (Carini 2001, p. 163). Clearly there are limits to solitary reflection and to learning alone.

The word 'team' appears in the title of this book. There are many views of it and many kinds of team. So Part Three of the book is devoted to clarifying this. For example, Brown and Bourne (1996) identify three levels of interdependence in teams. The integrated level where team members work together on a common task and where the effectiveness of one member is dependent on the others. The collaborative level where part of a workload may be shared and the independent level where team members work individually with little collaboration between them. The fundamental processes for developing reflective healthcare teams are collegial and public ones. This involves honest dedication to self-critique and continuous improvement and a willingness to take some risks when advocating for positive change. The two elements of risk and disclosure are also part of a process of changing the paradigm of change. For some the risks lie in naming problems and concerns which many would prefer to have left quiescent. In setting out this case, I am scaling up the practices of reflection so as to be a genuinely transformative approach to sustainable service development and to building better workplaces. A complex process indeed.

Facilitating reflection

Getting the most from reflection of one kind or another, often requires skilful facilitation. This may be provided from within the team or by someone external to it and the team's organisation. It is not uncommon for those who are reflecting on their practice to experience a level of discomfort when sharing personal experiences and particularly any associated painful or conflicting feelings. We should never forget that, for some, these feelings can be overwhelming. It is important therefore that all participants are aware that some forms of reflection come with a health warning! When a team gets together to learn through reflection many tensions can reveal themselves. Common ones are around attitudes towards things and people and particularly around self-belief. For example, there can be tensions between the 'will/will not' attitudes of team members and the 'can/cannot' people in the team. Figure 3.1 shows this.

Barker (2002) suggests that the 'will-can' people are to be prized and nurtured in every team. They may not only be 'willing horses' but highly competent ones also. In preparing for this book, I have met a number of 'willing-but-cannot' people. The 'cannot' dimension always seems to have two sides to it. One is about staff who feel they cannot move forward. It is a feeling from within them. The other is born out of an experience that there are systems, structures and influences that actively

	WILL	WILL NOT
CAN	Able to and ...	Sceptic
CANNOT	Willing to but ...	Troubled

Fig 3.1 Some tensions within a team.

work against staff moving forward. The sources of these are exterior to the team and individual. The sceptics in teams may be those who 'will not, but can'. This may mean that they will not act today but they may act in the future. All teams need sceptics. It is important that we are constructively sceptical. This is part of the critical being I described earlier. Without sceptics we may open ourselves up to the problems of groupthink. Teams with 'will not and cannot' members could be described as 'troubled teams' and potentially troublesome!

The practices of team reflection can make tensions like these more visible. The process therefore needs very careful and skilled facilitation. A crucial task of any facilitator is to try to link feelings and thinking to participant 'systems of relevance'. These might be:

- *Personal relevance.* For example, concerned with developing greater self-knowledge, self-understanding, self-belief, self-efficacy and so on.
- *Professional relevance.* For example, improving what is done with and for others such as patients, clients, carers and colleagues.
- *Political relevance.* For example, action that responds to policy imperatives and also (micro-political) action that can free us from unquestioning adherence to habitual routines, tradition, precedent, coercion, self-deception and so on.

I did not begin this section (The Reflective Lens) by asking, 'What is reflection and reflective practice?' but rather 'What are the interests of the practices of reflection?' This is a way to explore its values and purposes. I see reflection as being about our ability to move forward. However, we need to be clear that there is moving forward *by* oneself (or together with others) and *for* oneself (or for the team). Another important starting point then is to appreciate that the interests of reflection have been buffeted by, and have responded to, different influences over time. Recently, there has been a growth in the diversity of the purposes of reflection and in ways to engage with them. This has been a consequence of increasing organisational expectations of the practices of reflection to produce some kind of tangible gains or improvements in services. A further starting point for this book therefore is to engage in some re-thinking about customary conceptions and emerging interests of reflection. I list the essence of this re-thinking briefly now in order to draw upon it in more detail later (Part Two). I suggest that in intelligent, twenty-first century healthcare settings, four emergent interests of reflection, in the area of human life-work, are increasingly those of an interest in:

- *Being human-well.* With human well-being and being human, well.
- *Embracing uncertainty.* Working with fuzziness and at the creative edge of order and chaos.
- *The bottom line.* Not only with reflective skills and techniques but the way the practices of reflection need to be about delivering against

agreed targets and expectations. In other words to be more closely linked with evidence and results.

- *Asking serious questions*. Moving beyond, but not forgetting, Schön and Dewey.

I am not suggesting for a moment that these represent a new kind of consensus or orthodoxy, but more a diversity of interests symptomatic of at least three trends. First, services will be subjected to an annual 'health check' (replacing the star ratings system) and recently introduced by the Healthcare Commission in the UK. These checks will cover performance in the areas of safety, clinical and cost-effectiveness, governance, patient focus, accessible and responsive care, the care environment and amenities and public health. Second, these are changes in the nature of interactions between professionals (as providers) and the public (as consumers) of health and social care services. This trend is particularly noticeable in the positioning of service users 'front and central'. It provides opportunities to collectively reflect upon, and positively respond to, the things that really matter to patients and clients (Hanzak 2005). A third trend is change in the definition of 'skill' and vision of a skilled workforce (Block 1990, DoH 2002a, RCN 2003), a general shift in employer definitions of individual competence and a slow dismantling of hierarchical healthcare organisations into flatter and more team-based ones.

Taken collectively we can see subtle but important changes that emphasise the need for staff to have good personal and social skills, as well as the 'know-how' needed to discharge their role with care, safety and confidence. At least among 'core' staff, there are increasing expectations that they are able to work in a rapidly changing healthcare environment. Additionally staff are expected to engage in rule and policy making not only in rule and policy following behaviours and to work in multi-disciplinary teams. In short, increasing organisational efficiency is being seen to depend on the patterns and quality of communication, negotiation, influence and team work. These changes are as much a social as a technical issue, subject to vested interests and social conflict.

Chapter 4

Through the team lens

Investing in teams

Bourdieu (1997) asserts that the social world we inhabit is a world of accumulated history. He uses the notion of *capital* and its accumulation to bring this view to life. For him, capital is accumulated labour and is of different kinds. The application of two kinds, namely cultural and social capital, provides important starting points for this book. First, the *embodied state* of cultural capital helps us understand the functioning of individuals within a team in important ways. The embodied state is about dispositions of the mind and body. Capital accumulation assumes processes of embodiment, incorporation and acquisition which take time and which we must invest in personally. A positive sense of investment is important. Investment can take many forms. For example it may be in terms of attendance at a skills up-date day, an award-bearing course or in terms of an emotional investment in something personally significant. Investment and acquisition are about working on something and bettering oneself. In essence it is about self-improvement. Self-reflection fits in here as this kind of reflection can help bring about different kinds of improvement, particularly when linked with self-confidence, self-concept, self-worth, self-efficacy and so on.

Social capital on the other hand is essentially made up of social obligations, exchanges between staff, commitments and loyalties to others. It is therefore about relationships of mutual acquaintance and recognition. It is also about membership of a team and so provides members with the backing of the collectively-owned social capital. The amount of social capital possessed by a team thus depends upon the size and nature of the connections between members that can effectively be mobilised. Accumulating social capital is again a product of investment, individual and collective, conscious and unconscious. So we should see teams as possessing different kinds and amounts of capital, which when exchanged, can be used for material gain, professional satisfaction and personal pleasure. This capital can be used to form necessary and significant relationships that are subjectively felt by all team members in terms of feelings of togetherness, belonging, cohesion, gratitude, mutual respect, trust and friendship, for example. So the use of cultural and social capital forms, informs and can sustain teams. Standards for acceptable and preferred uses of capital define the team, its identity and capability. Exchanges affirm and reaffirm the work of its members. So when we say we are investing in the development of teams, we are also making a practical capital investment!

Trust in teams

A pervasive theme that runs through the literatures on service modernisation and workplace transformation is the importance of trust (Rogers 1995a, Rogers 1995b, Weber 1998, Fairholm & Fairholm 2000, Costa *et al.* 2001, Hupcey *et al.* 2001, Webber 2002, Costa 2003, Fichman 2003). Interestingly, because it is so widely acknowledged as essential we rarely probe more than superficially into its meaning and nature in practice. Because of this we are in danger of tuning it into a kind of 'black box' full of individual meanings. In the work described in Parts Three and Four of this book, trust certainly has at least two defining attributes. It appears to exist when team members find one another's thinking and actions reasonably predictable and where members share, substantially, the same values and team goals. Trust certainly illuminates our understanding of team dynamics and interpersonal relationships in certain contexts. But what about trust in healthcare settings where team membership and interpersonal relationships are much less stable and predictable over time? Giddens (1990, p. 34) offers us some kind of general starting point when he defines trust thus, 'Trust may be defined as confidence in the reliability of a person or system, regarding a given set of outcomes or events, where that confidence expresses a faith in the probity or love of another, or in the correctness of abstract principles'. So to paraphrase, we can place our trust in people or processes. For some this poses a dilemma. You may not see these as mutually exclusive. Maybe the dilemma can be stated as choosing to invest in the qualities and capabilities of team members or in the performance of systems? But they may need each other to function well!

Fundamental to reflective practices, in any context, is a feeling of trust and particularly trusting behaviours. Trust affects the pattern of relationships within and beyond teams. It also affects a team's ability to think and act differently. 'Mutual trust is a virtuous circle of anticipation and action whose initiation always requires a leap of faith beyond the available evidence' (Schön & Rein 1994, p. 179). But we often have to take risks to trust. Reflection for improvements in practice, policy and the workplaces, in which both are embedded, is not a risk-free business. We need to appreciate that there is a reciprocal relationship between trust and risk. Maister *et al.* (2002) offer six important insights on trust, which serve as important starting points for this book. In essence they are:

- *Trust grows.* Trust rarely develops instantly and does not happen without work, without volition, or without effort. It does not happen by magic.
- *Trust is emotional.* We value colleagues we can trust. Knowing we can trust them helps us feel good. Additionally, patients, clients and

their families place their trust in us. They trust our expertise and our dedication to serving their best interests.

- *Trust is a two-way relationship.* There are always things we can do to become more trustworthy. This may be to do with what we say and how we behave. But we do not have the ability to create both an atmosphere of trust and trusting behaviours on our own. Those we work with and for must also participate in this process and reciprocate appropriately.

- *Trust entails risk.* Trust without risk is a bit like lemonade without any fizz! The potential of trust violation is always there in a trusting relationship. After taking a while to develop, trust can evaporate in an instant. Who we trust and what we trust them with, can be a risky business.

- *Trust is experienced differently.* We can see trust as one person doing the trusting and one being trusted. These are different roles in the trust process. In reality the roles are not often as distinct as this. More subtly just because we feel we can trust does not mean we can be trusted. Maister *et al.* (2002) say, if we are incapable of trusting, we probably cannot be trusted.

- *Trust is personal.* Who can we trust in our workplaces? What do we place our trust in? Do we trust ourselves, our line manager, the CEO, the Board? How far can we place our trust in organisational processes such as those of resource allocation and decision-making? Building reflective teams requires that members place their trust in the principles and practices of reflection as well as in one another. A fundamental starting point in this book is a belief that trust is about relationships and reciprocity. These evidence themselves as shared values, expressed and lived out. They might be phrased thus. 'I know I can trust you to do the best you can. You can trust me to play my part and I acknowledge that our relationship is built on this shared value.'

Bevington *et al.* (2004, p. 28) talk about the importance of soft intelligence and do so particularly in relation to trusting people. They quote one UK strategic health authority chief executive, 'A lot of soft intelligence is about relationships and the test of any relationship is when things go wrong. If people invest enough time and effort in building relationships in the good times, when difficulties do arise there is a history of trust'. Linking with earlier points, another chief executive states that self-aware chief executives ' ... *are people who invest time and effort in reflecting on their practice, with help. In their interactions with me or key others, they demonstrate a trusting and open approach. You see how they react to different situations: do they call on their networks for advice and support, or curl up and hide away?'* (Bevington *et al.* 2004, p. 29).

Patterns of relationships

Understanding patterns of relationships is a fundamental organising idea for this book. I link it in Part Four with the notion of team wellness. In healthcare settings patterns manifest themselves in three important ways. First, they are to be found in the language(s) we use with each other and with those we care for. Second, in the patterns of interaction between staff of different grades and in different disciplines and between professionals and service users. Third, they manifest themselves in the feelings we experience in trying to initiate, develop and sustain humanly significant and caring relationships.

The Mobius Model (Demarest *et al.* 2004) is very helpful and interesting in its description of patterns of human relationships. It focuses on the role of conversation in impeding and developing relationships. Six essential qualities of relationships were identified in developing the Mobius model. They provide valuable starting points for issues I will discuss later in the book. Their qualities are:

- *Mutual understanding*, which exists when each person feels understood and also understands others. This is not the same as agreement. We may understand others in the workplace without necessarily agreeing with them.
- *Possibility* exists when those we work with and for become aware that thinking and acting differently is necessary and desirable if we are to realistically and positively move forward.
- *Commitment* exists when there is an agreement about how best to move forward and to achieve something worthwhile. Commitment is significantly influenced by personal and collective values and the exigencies of current practice.
- *Capability* is about ways to fulfil commitments to which everyone has agreed.
- *Responsibility* concerns agreement over what each person in the team will do to carry out their commitments.
- *Acknowledgements* exist when there is mutual recognition of what has been accomplished and what is still missing for the agreed commitments to be fully achieved. (Demarest *et al.* 2004, p. 5)

Plsek *et al.* (2004) argue that much of our change effort in the National Health Service in the UK is focused on structures that involve changing organisational boundaries, the deployment of resources, introducing new jobs, tools, targets and so on. They posit that we have learned many times over, in past change efforts, that modifying structures alone is probably not sufficient to bring about the transformations we seek, especially in complex systems like healthcare organisations. To truly bring about fundamental transformation in complex systems, they say that we also need to recognise the importance of patterns that drive thinking, learning and behaviour. By patterns they mean such things as patterns of power, decision-making and how various groups communicate with one another. They argue that failure to achieve fundamental change through re-organisation, re-engineering and re-design often lies in the fact that the underlying patterns in the system remain unchanged and unchallenged (Plsek *et al.* 2004, p. 3). Maybe what is also missing in this analysis is another word with 're' in it, namely reflection. One consequence of reflections of different kinds, that are appropriately recorded, is that they enable individuals, teams and organisations to develop a memory (DoH 2000). This provides opportunities for not only learning from inappropriate patterns of relationships but also opportunities for being proactive and preventing them happening in the first place.

Power and politics

The notion of individualism and the more general criticisms that reflective practices have been overly personal, apolitical and 'localist', are not the only starting points for this book. Another is that reflective practices have often failed to engage with issues of power and politics. Because of this, reflective practices have been reduced, by some, to a series of tools and techniques. This is a very impoverished view of the field, especially if you believe that learning through reflection is about positively transforming something of 'concern' in a healthcare setting.

We reflect in, through and on practice for a reason. It is an intentional activity. One pervasive intention is to change something. Another is to try to understand if this change, say in practice, might also constitute some kind of practice improvement. This process can be triggered by asking a question such as, 'How can I/we improve my/our practice here?' (Whitehead 1993). This question invites us to reflect on our current situation and how it has come to be the way it is. It is also an invitation to engage with issues of power and politics (to mention but two) as they are known, experienced, (re)produced and circulate between individuals, staff groups and teams. We ignore them at our peril, especially with UK government statements and intentions to 'shift the balance of power' within the health service (DoH 2002d). The power of individuals to change and improve health practice and policy is tied into broader systems of power relations through which individuals, teams and organisations are structurally (dis)empowered. Clearly politics and power matter. At the very least, reflective practices need to capture a more political sense of collective human agency. They also need to address the way cultures of power that exist within and between healthcare teams, disciplines and organisations, help or hinder improvement efforts.

There are at least five aspects to this that are relevant to this book. I list them briefly here.

- Power is enacted within teams through what people say and do.
- There are codes or rules for participating effectively in the power-play within and between teams. Codes and rules for example about how we present ourselves to others, the languages we use, what and how we write.
- These rules often say important things about the personal and professional qualities of those who have (or feel they have) formulated them.
- To participate effectively you have to know or be told the rules or codes. Without this knowledge we may hear ourselves saying 'Why don't they say what they mean?' or 'What's wrong with them, why don't they understand?' and so on.
- Strangely, we sometimes find that those with power are the ones least aware of, or least willing to acknowledge, its existence. For some an admission of this kind might be distinctly uncomfortable. For others it may be a force for alienation, loneliness and being apart from, rather than a part of, the team. Interestingly I have found that those with less power are often most aware of its existence and how it affects them.

A process of transformation

Developing reflective healthcare teams brings with it a strong sense that it is a process of transformation, in three senses of the word. The first is to do with transforming existing social relations between staff. Better team learning, team working and development is about transforming existing patterns of relationships. We need to understand and work with these patterns. Second, building reflective teams can involve transforming existing work practices. This is essentially about thinking and acting differently. Third, it often involves transforming organisational infrastructures so that creating and sustaining more team-based working is possible. So further starting points are views of transformation that embrace participation in reflective practices as a personal right and operating at individual, team and organisational levels.

A caveat ... no silver bullet cures

In times of major system failures we often hear senior personnel saying that it is 'now a time for deep reflection to ensure that this does not happen again'. Here reflection is in a reactive role. It is a process of trying to 'fix' things when they have gone wrong. It is also perceived by some as a kind of antidote to constant operational fire-fighting and crisis management. Reflective teams and reflective practices are not silver bullets! They do not and cannot cure all ills. So a final starting point is to assert that developing reflective teams needs to be part of a bigger process, that of building reflective healthcare organisations (Ghaye, Forthcoming). Some characteristics of such organisations are that they have a pervasive curiosity and an eagerness to learn more about themselves, how they are performing, how they are perceived by stakeholders and what might be improved within them. In such organisations reflection is both a catalyst for learning and a response to learning. Reflective practices are both proactive and reactive. Reflection helps fuel a culture of inquiry. Reflective teams are important attributes of such inquiring organisations. The practices of reflection are valued and sustained. The team and its practices make a significant contribution to the pervasive culture within the organisation.

References

Adams, R. (1990) *Self-help, Social Work and Empowerment*. Macmillan, Basingstoke.

Alvesson, M. (2003) *Understanding Organisational Culture*. Sage, London.

Barker, A. (2002) *The Alchemy of Innovation*. Spiro Press, London.

Barnett, R. (1997) *Higher Education: A Critical Business*. The Society for Research into Higher Education & The Open University, Buckingham.

Bevington, J., Stanton, P. & Cullen, R. (2004) Gently does it. *Health Service Journal*, 11 November.

Bevington, J. (2005) The Bevington Brief. *The Health Services Journal*, 6 January, 30.

Bleakley, A. (2000) Writing with invisible ink: narrative, confessionalism and reflective practice. *Reflective Practice* 1(1), 11–24.

Block, F. (1990) *Post-industrial Possibilities: A Critique of Economic Discourse*. University of California Press, Berkeley.

Block, P. (2002) *The Answer to How is Yes*. Berrett-Koehler, San Francisco.

Bolton, G. (2001) *Reflective Practice: Writing and Professional Development*. Paul Chapman Publishing, London.

Boud, D. & Walker, D. (1990) Making the most of experience. *Studies in Continuing Education* 12(2), 61–80.

Boud, D., Keogh, R. & Walker, D. (1993) *Using Experience for Learning*. SRHE and Open University Press, Buckingham.

Bourdieu, P. (1997) The forms of capital. In *Education, Culture, Economy, Society* (eds A. Halsey *et al.*). Oxford University Press, Oxford.

Brookfield, S. (1995) *Developing Critical Thinkers: Challenging Adults to Explore Alternative Ways of Thinking and Acting*. The Open University Press, Buckingham.

Brookfield, S. (2000a) The concept of critically reflective practice. In *Handbook of Adult and Continuing Education* (eds A. L. Wilson & E.R. Hayes). Jossey-Bass, San Francisco.

Brookfield, S. (2000b) Transformative learning as ideology critique. In *Learning as Transformation: Critical Perspectives on a Theory in Progress* (J. Mezirow & Associates). Jossey-Bass, San Francisco.

Brown, A. & Bourne, I. (1996) *The Social Work Supervisor*. Open University Press, Buckingham.

Burns, S. & Bulman, C. (2001) *Reflective Practice in Nursing: The Growth of the Professional Practitioner*. Blackwell Science, Oxford.

Carr, W. & Kemmis, S. (1986) *Becoming Critical: Education, Knowledge and Action Research*. The Falmer Press, Lewes.

Carini, P. (2001) *Starting Strong: A Different Look at Children, Schools and Standards*. Teachers College Press, New York.

Costa, A.C., Roe, R.A. & Taillieu, T. (2001) Trust within teams: the relation with performance effectiveness. *European Journal of Work and Organizational Psychology* **10** (3), 225–244.

Costa, A.C. (2003) Work team trust and effectiveness. *Personnel Review* **32**(5), 605–622.

Day, C., Elliott, J., Somekh, B. & Winter, R. (eds) (2002) *Theory and Practice in Action Research: Some International Perspectives*. Symposium Books, Oxford.

Demarest, L., Herdes, M., Stockton, J. & Stockton, W. (2004) *The Mobius Model: A Guide for Developing Effective Relationships in Groups, Teams and Organisations*. Farrar & Associates, Minneapolis.

Department of Health (2000) *An Organisation with a Memory*. DoH, London.

Department of Health (2001a) *Improving Working Lives for Doctors*. DoH, London.

Department of Health (2001b) *National Service Framework for Older People*. DoH, London.

Department of Health (2002a) *HR in the NHS Plan*. A document produced by the National Workforce Taskforce and HR Directorate for consultation. HMSO, London.

Department of Health (2002b) *Liberating the Talents: Helping Primary Care Trusts and Nurses to Deliver the NHS Plan*. DoH, London.

Department of Health (2002c) *Managing Excellence in the NHS*. DoH, London.

Department of Health (2002d) *Shifting the Balance of Power: The Next Steps*. DoH, London.

Department of Health (2004b) *Delivering HR in the NHS Plan: More Staff Working Differently*. DoH, London.

Department of Health (2004c) *Improving Hospital Doctors' Working Lives*. DoH, London.

Dewey, J. (1916) *Democracy and Education*. The Free Press, New York.

Drucker, P. (1985) *Innovation and Entrepreneurship*. Heinemann, London.

Fairholm, M. R. & Fairholm, G. (2000) Leadership amid the constraints of trust. *Leadership and Organization Development Journal* **21**(2), 102–109.

Fay, B. (1987) *Critical Social Science*. Cornell University Press, Ithaca.

Fichman, M. (2003) Straining towards trust: some constraints on studying trust in organizations. *Journal of Organizational Behaviour* **24**, 133–157.

Foucault, M. (1977) *Discipline and Punish*. Tavistock, London.

Freire, A.M.A. & Macedo, D. (1998) *The Paulo Freire Reader*. Continuum, New York.

Freire, P. (1972) *Pedagogy of the Oppressed*. Sheed and Ward, London.

Freire, P. (1974) *Education for Critical Consciousness*. Sheed and Ward, London.

Freire, P. (1994) *Pedagogy of Hope*. Continuum, New York.

Freire, P. (1998) *Pedagogy of the Heart*. Continuum, New York.

Ghaye, T. & Wakefield, P. (eds) (1993) *C.A.R.N. Critical Conversations: A Trilogy. Book One: The Role of Self in Action Research*. Hyde, Bournemouth.

Ghaye, T. (ed) (1995) *Creating Cultures for Improvement: Dialogues, Decisions and Dilemmas, Collaborative Action Research Network Critical Conversations: A Trilogy*. Hyde, Bournemouth.

Ghaye, T. & Ghaye, K. (1998) *Teaching and Learning through Critical Reflective Practice*. David Fulton, London.

Ghaye, T (Forthcoming) *Developing the Reflective Healthcare Organisation*. Blackwell Science, Oxford.

Giddens, A. (1990) *The Consequences of Modernity*. Polity Press, Oxford.

Glaze, J. (2002) PhD study and the use of a reflective diary: a dialogue with self. *Reflective Practice* **3**(2), 153–166.

Griffiths, M. (1998) *Educational Research for Social Justice: Getting Off the Fence*. Open University Press, Milton Keynes.

Groesbeck, R. & van Aken, E. M (2001) Enabling team wellness: monitoring and maintaining teams after start-up. *Team Performance Management* **7**(1/2), 11–20.

Gully, T. (2004) Reflective writing as critical reflection in work with sexually abusive adolescents. *Reflective Practice* **5**(3), 313–326.

Habermas, J. (1977) Hannah Arendt's communications concept of power. *Social Research* **44**(1), 3–24.

Hanzak, E. (2005) The things that really matter to patients. *Professional Nurse* **20**(5), 6.

Hupcey, J.E., Penrod, J., Morse, J.M. & Mitcham, C. (2001) An exploration and advancement of the concept of trust. *Journal of Advanced Nursing* **36**(2), 282–293.

Jack, R. (ed) (1995) *Empowerment in Community Care*. Chapman and Hall, London.

Johns, C (2000) *Becoming a Reflective Practitioner*. Blackwell Science, Oxford.

Johns, C. & Freshwater, D. (eds) (1998) *Transforming Nursing Through Reflective Practice*. Blackwell Science, Oxford.

Johns, C. (2002) *Guided Reflection: Advancing Practice*. Blackwell Science, Oxford.

Johnson, R. & Redmond, D. (1998) *The Art of Empowerment*. Pitman, London.

Joyce, W., Nohria, N. & Roberson, B. (2003) *What Really Works: The 4 + 2 Formula for Sustained Business Success*. Harper Business, New York.

Keiffer, C. (1984) Citizen empowerment: a developmental perspective. *Prevention in Human Services* **3**, 9–36.

Kember, D. *et al.* (2001) *Reflective Teaching and Learning in the Health Professions*. Blackwell Science, Oxford.

Kendall, S. (1998) *Health and Empowerment: Research and Practice*. Arnold, London.

Krmpotić-Schwind, J. (2003) Reflective process in the study of illness stories as experienced by three nurse teachers. *Reflective Practice* **4**(1), 19–32.

Kur, E. (1996) The faces model of high performing team development. *Management Development Review* **9**(6), 25–35.

Lander, D. & English, L.M. (2000) Doing research 'with': reading and writing our difference. *Reflective Practice* **1**(3), 343–358.

Latter, S. (1998) Health promotion in the acute setting: the case of empowering nurses. In *Health and Empowerment: Research and Practice* (ed. S. Kendall). Arnold, London.

Le May, A. (1998) Communication skills. In *Nursing Elderly People* (eds S. Redfern & F. Ross). Harcourt Brace, Edinburgh.

LePage, P. & Sockett, H. (2002) *Educational Controversies: Toward a Discourse of Reconciliation*. Routledge Falmer, London.

Livsey, R., & Palmer, P.J. (1999) *The Courage to Teach: A Guide to Reflection and Renewal*. Jossey-Bass, San Fransisco.

Longnecker, R. (2002) The jotter wallet: invoking reflective practice in a family practice residency program. *Reflective Practice* **3**(2), 219–224.

Loo, R. & Thorpe, K. (2002) Using reflective learning journals to improve individual and team performance. *Team Performance Management: An International Journal* **8**(5/6), 134–139.

Luke, A. (2004) Two takes on the critical. In *Critical Pedagogies and Language Learning* (eds B. Norton & K. Toohey). Cambridge University Press, Cambridge.

Luke, S. (1974) *Power: A Radical View*. Macmillan, London.

Maister, D., Green, C. & Galford, R. (2002) *The Trusted Advisor*. Simon & Schuster UK, London.

Martin, R. (2003) *The Responsibility Virus*. Basic Books, New York.

Marton, F. & Booth, S. (1997) *Learning and Awareness*. Lawrence Erlbaum Associates, New Jersey.

McCormack, B. (2001) 'The dangers of missing a chapter': a journey of discovery through reflective academic study. *Reflective Practice* **2**(2), 209–219.

Moon, J. (2004) *A Handbook of Reflective and Experiential Learning: Theory and Practice*. RoutledgeFalmer, London.

Morss, J. (1996) *Growing Critical: Alternatives to Developmental Psychology*. Routledge, London.

Parker, S. (1997) *Reflective Teaching in the Postmodern World: A Manifesto for Education in Postmodernity*. Open University Press, Buckingham.

Piper, S. & Brown, P. (1998) Psychology as a theoretical foundation for health education in nursing; empowerment or social control? *Nurse Education Today* **18**, 637–41.

Plsek, P., Bibby, J. & Garrett, S. (2004) *Mapping Behavioural Patterns: Exploring the Underlying Factors that Accelerate or Impede System Transformation*. NHS Modernisation Agency, London.

Pollard, A. & Tann, S. (1994) *Reflective Teaching in the Primary School: A Handbook for the Classroom*. Cassell, London.

Rainbow, P. (ed.) (1991) *The Foucault Reader*. Penguin, London.

Reason, P. & Bradbury, H. (eds) (2001) *Handbook of Action Research: Participative Inquiry & Practice*. Sage, London.

Reina, D., & Reina, M. (1999) *Trust and Betrayal in the Workplace*. Berrett-Koehler, San Francisco.

Reynolds, M. & Vince, R. (eds) (2004) *Organizing Reflection*. Ashgate, Aldershot.

Risner, D. (2002) Motion and marking in reflective practice: artifacts, autobiographical narrative and sexuality. *Reflective Practice* **3**(1), 5–19.

Rogers, R.W. (1995a) The psychological contract of trust – Part 1. *Executive Development* **8**(1), 15–19.

Rogers, R.W. (1995b) The psychological contract of trust – Part 2. *Executive Development* **8**(2), 7–15.

Rolfe, G., Freshwater, D. & Jasper, M. (2001) *Critical Reflection for Nursing and the Helping Professions: A User's Guide*. Palgrave, Basingstoke.

Royal College of Nursing (2003) *The Future Nurse : The RCN Vision*. RCN, London.

Ryles, S. (1999) A concept analysis of empowerment: its relationship to mental health nursing. *Journal of Advanced Nursing* **29**(3), 600–607.

Schön, D. & Rein, M. (1994) *Frame Reflection: Towards the Resolution of Intractable Policy Controversies*. Basic Books, New York.

Schön, D. (1998) *The Reflective Practitioner: How Professionals Think in Action*. Ashgate, Brookfield.

Sheard, A. & Kakabadse, A. (2002) Loose groups to effective teams: the nine key factors of the team landscape. *Journal of Management Development* **21**(2), 133–151.

Shepherd, M. (2004) Reflections on developing a reflective journal as a management adviser. *Reflective Practice* **5**(2), 199–208.

Siegel, H. (1988) *Educating Reason*. Routledge & Kegan Paul, London.

Slife, B. & Williams, R. (1995) *What's Behind the Research? Discovering Hidden Assumptions in the Behavioural Sciences*. Sage, London.

Stapleton-Watson, J. & Wilcox, S. (2000) Reading for understanding: methods of reflecting on practice. *Reflective Practice* **1**(1), 57–67.

Stuart, C.C. (2001) The reflective journeys of a midwifery tutor and her students. *Reflective Practice* **2**(2), 171–184.

Taylor, B. (2000) *Reflective Practice: A Guide for Nurses and Midwives*. Open University Press, Buckingham.

Taylor, I. (1997) *Developing Learning in Professional Education: Partnerships for Practice*. SRHE and Open University Press, Buckingham.

Thorpe, K (2004) Reflective learning journals: from concept to practice. *Reflective Practice* 5(3), 327–343.

Tones, K. (1993) The theory of health promotion: implications for nursing. In *Research in Health Promotion and Nursing* (eds J. Wilson-Barnett & C. Macleod). Macmillan, Basingstoke.

Tsang, W.K. (2003) Journaling from internship to practice teaching. *Reflective Practice* 4(2), 221–240.

Tuckman, B.W. (1965) Development sequence in small groups. *Psychological Bulletin* **63**, 384–399.

Tuckman, B.W. & Jenson, M.A. (1977) Stages of small group development revisited. *Group and Organization Studies* **2**, 419–427.

Velody, I. & Williams, R. (eds) (1998) *The Politics of Constructionism*. Sage, London.

von Krogh, G., Ichijo, K. & Nonaka, I. (2000) *Enabling Knowledge Creation: How to Unlock the Mystery of Tacit Knowledge and Release the Power of Innovation*. Oxford University Press, Oxford.

Webber, S.S. (2002) Leadership and trust facilitating cross-functional team success. *Journal of Management Development* **21**(3), 201–214.

Weber, L.R. (1998) On constructing trust: temporality, self-disclosure & perspective taking. *International Journal of Sociology and Social Policy* **18**(1), 7–26.

Winter, R. & Munn-Giddings, C. (2001) *A Handbook for Action Research in Health and Social Care*. Routledge, London.

Whitehead, J. (1993) *The Growth of Educational Knowledge: Creating Your Own Living Educational Theories*. Hyde, Bournemouth.

Zuber-Skerritt, O. (ed) (1996) *New Directions in Action Research*. The Falmer Press, Lewes.

Part Two

About REFLECTION: Learning through its interests and practices

Chapter 5
Reflecting on practice

So how can we *'develop reflective healthcare teams that are able to sustain high quality, personalised care?'* A first step is to find something significant to reflect on. Second, we need to find a medium through which to learn well. I want to suggest that scenario-based learning is such a medium. Errington's (2003, p. 10) view of a scenario is that they, '... may constitute a set of circumstances, a description of human behaviour, an outline of events, a story of human endeavour, an incident within a professional setting, a human dilemma/problem/issue and/or any other means that focuses on the interactions of humans with each other and their world'. Errington makes the point that reflecting on different kinds of scenario enables us to learn better. The general point I am making is that when we reflect, and in different ways, we have to reflect *on* something. For teams it is important that we agree what that something is!

A 'lived-experience' scenario: a tale from a maternity unit

Mrs Padda, of Indian origin, has made a complaint about the maternity unit where she had her baby. Her concerns were about her perceived lack of personalised, responsive care throughout her pregnancy, childbirth and postnatal period. You come to hear about some of her experiences. Here are two examples.

- Mrs Padda feels that throughout her pregnancy midwives did not give her time to properly take in what they were saying and that they didn't give her a chance to ask questions. They did not seem to recognise her personal needs, rather, certain assumptions were made because, Mrs Padda alleges, of her ethnic background. Particular offence was caused by one midwife's assumption that she wanted a son. Comments to this effect were made several times.
- Mrs Padda also complains that care in labour was fragmented, provided by several midwives whom she had not met before, who seemed to have several women to care for and who left her alone for long periods of time. Mrs Padda had felt frightened and was upset that her frequent request for pain relief, to one particular midwife, was ignored. Although she acknowledges that the midwives had not deliberately intended to be unkind, she asserts that they were not listening to her, or her sister-in-law who was supporting her.

It becomes known to you that similar complaints have been made before over the past two years and yet little improvement has occurred. The Head of Midwifery explains how the midwives feel over-worked and under-resourced and tells you that recruitment is notoriously difficult. She believes they are giving the very best care that they can, under chronically difficult circumstances. She says that in this instance, as safety was not compromised, there is nothing to be gained by scape-goating any one individual. She concludes by saying, 'We offer our sincere apologies to Mrs Padda and her husband. We are an extremely busy maternity unit'.

If we reflect on this scenario, there is much to learn. There are issues about human well-being. There are concerns and uncertainties, different understandings of the situation and staff trying to do the best they can. The scenario enables us to ask some serious questions about Mrs Padda's experience of giving birth in a particular maternity unit. Questions can be asked about how Mrs Padda's experience has come to be as she claims. The scenario also provides opportunities to explore whose interests are being served and in what ways. Reflecting on it also opens up possibilities for a conversation about areas for possible practice improvement. This is *reflection-for-action*, which should be:

- Informed: we are clear about why we are acting in a particular manner. This is action informed by our values.
- Committed: we are sure about what we are committed to try to do.
- Intentional: we are clear about what our intention is, what the purpose of our actions are.
- Sustainable: we not only plan to make particular interventions but also how to keep the action going to sustain success.

Learning through writing about practice: creating a 'text'

Within the field of the practices of reflection, writing (or creating a text) is generally an individualistic activity. Most often it is linked with journaling, the use of a diary, learning logs, portfolio building and award-bearing courses of one kind or another. Writing about practice on one's own is a challenge in itself. Engaging in some shared writing, amongst team members, can be even more challenging. Also, learning through reflections on what has been written is not as straightforward as many think. I include an extended list of good examples here that are drawn from medical education, social care, nursing, allied health, management learning, teaching, and pre- and post-registration contexts, which are very useful reading (Holly 1987, Purisky *et al.* 1998, Bolton 2001, Kember et al. 2001, Klemola & Norros 2001, MacFarlane 2001, Noble 2001, Maloney & Campbell-Evans 2002, Crawford *et al.* 2002, Vince 2002, Williams *et al.* 2002).

I am not going to attempt any kind of summary of these. Rather I want to draw your attention to an excellent paper written by Bleakley (2000), where the act of writing about what we feel, think and do is placed in a broader frame of 'narrative ways of knowing'. Simply put, this is the act of telling a kind of story. One view is that it is about reflecting on practice through a personal-confessional mode of writing. Bleakley offers a critique of writing in this genre and offers alternatives. Through writing over speaking as a medium for reflection on practice, Bleakley provocatively explores the claims made that writing should not be linked, uncritically, to ideas of personal growth and development. He enables us to see behind the obvious. For example, '... tumours grow, economies inflate, obesity is growth... growth is usually taken to mean expansion, differentiation, progress, synthesis, maturation (growing up) or becoming creative. Yet it can also be viewed as deepening (growing down), intensification, shedding, repetition, or emptying' (Bleakley 2000, p. 13). He questions overly simplistic descriptions of the context for such personal-confessional writing, like 'safe' and within a 'climate of trust' and cause-effect links between these and 'enhancing catharsis'.

Bleakley presents a view that sometimes the context for learning is 'dangerous', particularly when staff are questioning habitual patterns of thinking and practice. These are situations, '... of "danger", as in pointing out the unworthiness of established or normative practices that are unethical, hypocritical, unreflexive, congealing, or sloppy' (Bleakley 2000, p. 14). He advises that we should not privilege the personal-confessional mode at the expense of writing in other ways. There is some important progress being made to embrace this, for example in physiotherapy by Clouder (2000), Donaghy and Morss (2000) and in nursing ethics by Durgahee (1997b). In the light of all of this, perhaps we should reflect even more deeply on the contents of the Royal College of Nursing's statement about team working (note 'working' not 'learning'!). '*Good team working requires trust, commitment and respect. It also requires that the contribution of all members of the team, and the patients they serve, is valued. Teams need strong leadership and good channels of communication ...*' (RCN 2003, p. 22).

Three aspects of reflective writing that get much less exposure are to do with purposes, ethics and creative tensions.

Purposes

Ghaye and Lillyman (1998) assert that learning through reflective writing can serve many purposes. Purpose influences what is written, and how it is undertaken. For example, the writing can serve professional accountability and re-validation purposes, an evaluative purpose for aspects of practice, to facilitate critical thinking, to release feelings and frustrations, to see different 'truths' and develop better ways of 'noticing' (Mason 2002). I briefly elaborate seven purposes below. They are not mutually exclusive.

1 *Writing to record a team's experiences.* To be useful, these experiences need to be placed in a context, re-visited and re-read over time. A key question to ask is, 'So what are we learning?'
2 *Writing to enhance a team's understanding of practice.* This requires an interpretation of what is written. We can do this by reading what is written through different reflective lenses. For example, through re-lationships, decision-making, power, conflict, communication and participation lenses.
3 *Writing that enables a team to develop.* For some what is written fulfils a need to tell, to disclose and enter into dialogue with others around. This is what we did, for these reasons. This is what it felt like. These were the outcomes. So what do you think?
4 *Writing to demonstrate a team's competence and capability.* This reflects a need to be accountable and responsible for collective action, a desire to continuously improve practice and an acknowledgement that evidence is needed to demonstrate competence and capability.
5 *Writing to bring a sense of 'order' to turbulent practice settings.* Writing holds our practice still for a moment. A single piece of writing is frozen text waiting to be reflected upon. For a moment it brings a kind of order to things. Ackoff (1979) calls dynamic, turbulent and often chaotic situations 'messes'. Writing has the potential to help unravel the mess.
6 *Writing as a collective celebration.* Here the central purpose is to write about an aspect of practice that the team is proud of. The piece of writing acts as a tribute and something that depicts current 'best practice' or the best the team could do, in the circumstances.
7 *Writing to build on a team's success.* Writing can have a prospective quality and not simply be about past events. It can mark the beginning of an action plan to build on and sustain current success.

Ethics

There are two complex issues to consider. I set them out briefly here. They are about rights, risks and benefits (Durgahee 1997a, 1997b, Heath 1998, Molloy & Cribb 1999).

1 *The issue of rights.* Writing about practice involves self-respect, respect for others, esteem and dignity. Writers need to exercise their right to determine what is written about and in what way. Team members should not be coerced into making public what is written. They have the right to privacy. Members should be the ones who determine the time, extent and context under which they disclose what they have written to those outside the team. Having said this, there is always a possibility that what is written down may be subpoenaed. All writing about practice is situated within a context of litigation.
2 *The issue of risks and benefits.* Any kind of writing and reflection can generate feelings of discomfort and vulnerability. They can do harm. It is not always an inherently 'safe' activity. This may be the case if teams ask themselves questions like: Why is our clinical practice like

this? How did it come to be this way? How can we improve it? A team's commitment to learn through reflections on their practice, is a commitment to a great deal of introspection, honesty with self and others and a frame of mind that gives them a good chance of responding positively to what they come to know.

Creative tensions

Reflective writing and learning from it is a tensioned relationship. Four commonly experienced tensions are given here. Ghaye and Lillyman (1998) provide a more detailed list.

1   *Between writing personal and safe responses.* The former is about content. It concerns that which is significant to the team. The latter links the message with the medium. Sometimes safe responses are written in a context of fear, dread and blame. Sometimes they are written up so as not to offend if they were to enter the public domain in some way.

2   *Between team-centric views and the views of significant others.* This is about writing to present the team's view of things and staff's ability and preparedness to be open to the views of others. No account is free from bias and an amount of distortion (wilful or unconscious). No account is neutral, 'innocent' or impartial. In the context of greater public and patient involvement in health, alternative points of view on issues facing the team are important.

3   *Between privacy and the right to know.* This is a complex and very contested area. I have said that a team has the right to keep the contents of its reflective writing within the team, if staff so wish. However, this raises professional, moral, ethical and legal issues concerning the rights others have to know what it is the team may be writing about them. Rights are problematic because they often contain appeals to different political, professional and moral values (Pring 1988).

4   *Between the particular and the general.* One piece of writing can be an account of a particular instance of practice, an encounter, a dialogue, a feeling, an achievement, and so on. It is dangerous to read too much into one entry. Writing over time provides the potential for generalisation. This might be a generalisation about a personally preferred value position in relation to client care, about a general strategy for managing the busyness of a ward, and so on. In this sense 'general' means what a team tends to generally do, think and feel. It may or may not be generally true for others. It is important to appreciate the difference between what is generally the case for one team and what is not. Through conversation it is important to try to tease out what is particular and different in certain clinical contexts and what are the more patterned, regular and therefore more general things. If teams make these general things known to others, they give them the opportunity to generalise from them, to their own clinical situation. This is called naturalistic generalisation (Stake 1995).

Table 5.1   Scenario-building guidelines.

Brief-but-Vivid:	Try to write no more than a paragraph but in doing so, capture an event vividly
Understandable:	Others who were not there should be able to understand the event.
Discussable:	The scenario should raise something important to talk about.
Real:	It should be about a real 'lived' event, as experienced by someone (you with others).
Learning:	You should build in a number of things you feel need to be reflected upon.

When writing about practice it is important to reflect on the ordinary and successful aspects of a team's work and not just on the extra-ordin-ary/dramatic/traumatic/worrying and problematic aspects of it. The key is to find something a team is genuinely interested in and committed to trying to improve. The source of this might be something that made team members think during or after the event. Table 5.1 provides some general guidelines for scenario-building.

There is now a substantial body of knowledge that confirms that writing about practice and then reflecting on it in team meetings, can enhance team learning (Jay 1995, Clarke *et al.* 1996, Astor *et al.* 1998, White 1998, Zollo 1998, Soohbany 1999, Glover 2000, Paget 2001).

Time is always our enemy, but this practice may be worth a try. It provides an opportunity for a team to learn more about a substantive aspect of their clinical practice and the organisational cultures in which it is embedded. For example, a team might learn more about caring for the elderly, about how to maximise the therapeutic potential of nursing, the rights of the unborn child, effective multidisciplinary team leadership, and so on. Second, writing offers the opportunity to learn about the process of researching clinical practice, what questions to ask, what evidence to gather and what valid claims can be made about improvements in practice. Third, writing offers an opportunity to learn about ourselves, about the kind of healthcare professional we are and wish to be.

The interests and practices of reflection in the twenty-first century

Arguably many of the current practices of reflection have an interest in four major areas of human life-work. I offer them as a catalyst for further thinking and action, not as an absolute truth on the matter. There are no boundaries between the four areas of interest. Try to see them as *spaces* where I believe we find certain interests being expressed. The *spaces-between are spaces for creativity*. This space is ambiguous and therefore provides room for finding more of ourselves. In doing this we may be in a position to judge for ourselves whether we believe that, '... reflective practice has lost its way, that it has been reduced from a radical alternative to technical rationality into merely an adjunct to it, a tool to be applied in order to meet "the mandatory requirements for post-registration education" (DoH, 1999). This has entailed not only a loss of direction, but a loss of status, and, indeed, a loss of self-determination. Reflective practice no longer sets its own agenda but must take its rather lowly place within the hierarchy of nursing evidence where, judged according to the criteria of prevailing evidence-based paradigm, it is likely to attract little attention and even less funding ... sadly, most people no longer even question the dominant paradigm, being content instead to adapt their beliefs and practices to the prevailing hegemony. After all that's where all the money is' (Rolfe 2001, p. 28).

This is a provocative paper from Rolfe raising issues that, I suggest, everyone who is serious about practising reflection, needs to mull over and decide whether Rolfe has a point. It may even stir you in to action! A loss of direction and self-determination are serious suggestions. How far do you feel this is the case? Is it this, or a natural and necessary process of ongoing transformation and realignment? If Rolfe's suggestions are true, do we need to address them? Does this situation release new possibilities? No longer being able to set its own agenda may say more about those who profess to practise reflection than about reflection itself. For me the most depressing tale of all is encapsulated in Rolfe's phrase, '... *most people no longer even question the dominant paradigm*'. This of course may well be paradigms (plural) depending on where we are 'situated'. I will come back to some of these points later.

Currently four major and prevailing interests of the practices of reflection in the area of human life-work appear to be:

- *An interest in being-human-well*. The practices of reflection on the work of individuals and teams.
- *An interest in embracing uncertainty*. The practices of reflection as working with fuzziness and the challenges involved in service improvement and workplace transformation.
- *An interest in the bottom line*. The practices of reflection as improving practice and getting results.
- *An interest in asking 'serious questions'*. The practices of questioning habit, routine, custom and orthodoxy. This requires what Dewey (1933) called the emotional involvement of the practitioner and not just a cerebral one. This interest also involves individual and collective capabilities of criticality and creativity.

Chapter 6

An interest in being-human-well: the practices of reflection on the work of individuals and teams

In thinking about this 'interest' I have been greatly influenced by the work, in the field of ethics, of Böhme (2001). He describes being-human-well thus: 'The use of the adverb implies that this formulation does not refer to an attribute of the human being, but to a quality of being human. What is at issue, therefore, is not certain attributes which qualify as good, attributes which are traditionally called virtues, but an accomplishment, the accomplishment of being human. This implies that one can be what one is in any case, namely a human being, in different ways, and in particular, more or less well .... the attempt to be human well is not really a striving to achieve a goal, but rather an endeavour to engage fully in being human and to disown nothing which forms part of it' (Böhme, 2001, p 89). This conception raises the question: How far is being-human-well possible on one's own? Böhme has a view on this. He states, 'If being-human-well means really engaging with the human situation, and fully living what it is to be a human being, it soon becomes clear that the humanity of the human being cannot be fulfilled in isolation' (Böhme 2001, p. 94). But of course people are, and do live in isolation. Some are isolated spatially, physically and psychologically. Some are periphera-lised, marginalised, excluded and silenced.

I am not saying that this does not necessarily lead to a fulfilled life, as this rather violates the respect we owe others in their otherness and their choice, need and wish to preserve and develop their individuality. Creating life-chances so that we can be-a-part, '... implies openness and attentiveness towards that which one is or can be with another, and it also means exposing oneself to the other and being affected by what affects him or her' (Böhme 2001, p. 95). In the context of developing reflective healthcare teams, like many other contexts of team learning and working, this is not always easy. The act of 'exposing oneself to another' and 'being affected' presupposes many things. On the positive side it is connected to trusting, supportive and enabling relationships. On the potentially 'darker' side we find the interactions of power, micro-politics and truth at work. Everything I have just listed can be problematic for some teams. In healthcare, I would suggest, what is called for is at least a commitment to a value position that says that we refuse to evade the issues of openness and attentiveness to others. If we fail to do this we cannot claim to be open-minded in the Dewey (1933) sense. If we evade these, how far can we claim that we are being-human-well?

Central to what I am describing here is a view of the humanity of the person, which is infused by self-understandings (Watson 1999). It is about a heightened sense of one's being. In a pragmatic sense it has a relationship to the elaboration of human self-understanding. It is an awareness that the past is not irrelevant. History matters. It influences the present and helps to shape the future. It is also an appreciation that the self as knower and as known, is a consequence of an interactive relationship between the I/me's, (individualism) and the us/we's (collectivism). There is still a strong interest in the I/me's in the field of reflection. This interest is to be found in Schön's (1983) work on the reflective practitioner and in some more contemporary work, for example in work framed by reference to the (therapeutic) self and others that focuses essentially on self-study Johns and Freshwater 1998, Johns 2000a, 2001a, 2002, Stuart 2001, Higgs and Andresen 2001, McCormack 2001, Freshwater 2002).

Reflections on Schön

So what, in essence, did Schön say to make his work so pervasive? Why do his ideas command such interest and influence? There are three main reasons for this state of affairs. Schön disliked the dominant and prevailing way in which knowledge about and for practice was conceived. He mistrusted and disliked the way three things were being separated – he called them 'dichotomies'. In particular, the dichotomies were.

1   The way means were being separated from ends.
2   The way research was separated from practice.
3   The separation of knowing from doing.

   Schön not only argued against these three things but, in doing so, emphasised that we should recognise the importance of 'practical knowledge'. He disliked these three dichotomies so much that he said we should look for an alternative 'epistemology of practice'. In other words, that we should think about the way we generate and value knowledge in a very different way (Schön 1971).

Schön and his dislike of technical rationality

Schön's work contains a critique of 'technical rationality' (see Starting Points). This is linked to the idea of practice being separated from theory and of the 'worker' (such as the nurse, midwife, health visitor, therapist, social worker, doctor, and so on) being seen as a 'technician' who almost unthinkingly applies other people's knowledge to his or her own practice. Schön argued that the 'technical-rational' ways of viewing the links between the generation of knowledge and professional practice were (and still are?) dominant. Briefly, this means that knowledge is generated in and by 'elites', often based in universities and research centres. This knowledge is 'theoretical' and is about how to achieve certain 'ends'. Hospitals, homes that care for the elderly, units, wards, departments, surgeries, walk-in clinics and the like are worlds of practice. In this technical-rational mode of thinking, the healthcare workers' task is viewed as applying the theoretical knowledge from the universities or the 'academy', in order to solve their practical problems. It is an application of theory to practice, and it devalues the knowledge that clinicians, for example, develop about and through their work (Whitehead 1993). Clinicians are viewed as 'technicians' because they never question the values that underpin their practice and make them the kind of healthcare professionals they are. They rarely question the context in which they are working, and how this liberates or constrains what they do.

There are some very real problems incurred with holding this technical-rational view. First, the ends or products of healthcare work are rarely fixed. They are often contested. People have different views about them. This is pervasive in the caring and helping professions. Take any 'end' that you can think of – it does not have to be clinical in kind, it could be managerial or professional – and then reflect on this point. The 'ends' (as well as the means!) can be contested. Are the ends to 'make individuals feel better', 'to remedy clinical deficits', 'to provide management with a stick', or 'to help to foster a learning culture within the organisation', and so on, incontestable? Second, we need to question the usefulness and relevance of knowledge that is produced out of the context to which it is to be applied. We have to ask questions about who is generating this knowledge for practitioners, and what exactly their motives are. This separation of the knowledge 'producers' from the 'consumers' is seen by some as divisive and elitist. Hooks (1995, p. 64), for example, holds the following view of the situation: '... *the uses these individuals (i.e. academics) make of theory is instrumental. They use it to set up unnecessary and competing hierarchies of thought which re-inscribe the politics of domination by designing work as either inferior, superior, or more or less worthy of attention ... And it is easy to imagine different locations, spaces outside academic exchange, where such theory would not only be seen as useless, but as politically non-progressive, a kind of narcissistic, self-indulgent practice that at most seeks to create a gap between theory and practice so as to perpetuate class elitism'.*

A third difficulty with holding the technical-rational view is that the assumption that the problems of everyday clinical practice can always be solved by applying someone else's knowledge to one's own practice, is simplistic. It devalues the art and skilfulness of the healthcare professional caring for particular patients in particular circumstances. A team's everyday 'problems' are not simply pre-defined, but are constructed through engagement with the '... *indeterminate zone of practice which, typically, is characterised by uncertainty, uniqueness and value conflict'* (Schön 1987, p. 6).

So what does a team do when members find that, in trying to apply theory to practice, the theory fails to solve their immediate, local and particular concerns? What happens when the theory fails to explain the team's practice to them and to others? In the busy, fuzzy and often chaotic worlds of clinical practice, concerns are many and varied, often difficult to define and sometimes to resolve. They cannot always be solved by the application of someone else's theoretical knowledge. Schön turns this technical-rational view around and talks about how reflection helps us to 'frame' and 're-frame' problems; how we should value and use the kind of knowledge that is embedded in our workplaces, generated by our practice and shared amongst practitioners themselves. This set of issues is summed up by Gould (1996, pp. 2–3): 'A not uncommon illustration of this might be a duty social worker, called to the police station to assess someone arrested for a breach of the peace because the arresting officer thinks the person may be suffering from a mental disorder. Whether the professional social work issues raised by this situation relate primarily to criminality, a mental health crisis or some other problem still to be discovered such as homelessness, is not pre-determined at the point of referral, but is negotiated via a complex series of transactions between the worker, the detained individual and possibly other actors such as police or psychiatrists'.

From this perspective, the kind of 'theoretical' knowledge described is not neutral and value-free. For example, ' . . . *which can be drawn down and directly applied, but . . . only of use when mediated through the complex filters of practice experience. In order to become a tool for practice, the practitioner has to transform theory in the light of learning from past experience (reflection-on-action)*' (Gould, 1996, pp. 2–3).

Schön and joining up practice with theory

There are three elements in Schön's idea of practical knowledge. These are 'knowing-in-action', 'reflection-in-action' and 'reflection-on-practice'. I have also linked these with Argyris and Schön's (1992) helpful ideas of a 'theory-of-action' and 'knowing-in-action'.

Knowing-in-action linked to theories-of-action

The essence of this element, in Schön's view of practical knowledge, is that what we know shows in what we do. There are two parts to this. The first is that in trying to improve practice we have to begin by reflecting on what we actually do. This reflection generates a rich and detailed knowledge base. The second part is that this knowledge is drawn upon by us in our caring work. It then becomes our 'knowing-in-action'. Much of this knowing is often difficult to make explicit, to name and talk about. Schön

(1992) and others (Claxton 1999, Atkinson & Claxton, 2000) called it 'intuition' and 'instinct'. This view of knowing-in-action is linked to an extremely different view of theory from that described earlier. It is a view that acknowledges that we develop our own theories, 'customised' and 'tailored' ones, which help to guide and explain what we do. We have 'theories' about appropriate care management, about the best use of limited resources, about effective leadership, about communicating meaningfully, and so on. Making this kind of theory explicit, that is putting words to it and discussing it, is an important function of reflection.

Schön develops this idea in his work with Argyris (1992). They pull all of these thoughts together into their view of a 'theory-of-action'. This is a highly relevant collection of ideas and, again, comes in two parts – our 'espoused' theories and our 'theories-in-use'. The former is what we say or claim we do, even want to do. The latter is about what actually happens in practice. Normally we can find out what these theories-in-use are if we observe a colleague at work. Reflection provides the basis for improvement of our theories-in-use. We have a problem, though, if we cannot articulate what these theories are! Argyris and Schön (1992, p. 10) make the point, '*How can we change an existing theory-in-use or learn a new theory-in-use when we cannot state what is to be changed or learned?*'.

Reflection-in-action

When our 'knowing-in-action' produces an unexpected outcome or a surprise, one of two types of reflection can then follow, reflection-in-action and reflection-on-practice. The first is that which occurs during (but without interrupting) on-going work. What distinguishes reflection-in-action from other kinds of reflection is its immediate significance for action. It is thinking about how to reshape (and adjust) what we are doing whilst it is underway. Schön argued that it is central to the art by which professionals handle and resolve their difficulties and concerns *about* practice, whilst actually *in* practice. Essentially, it is about thinking in the midst of action. It is thinking about doing something whilst actually doing it. Thinking about what to say to a patient whilst saying it. Thinking about handling a conflict situation, such as needing to admit a patient on to a ward when there is no bed available, whilst actually trying to resolve it. It is not about 'stopping and thinking' in the midst of action. It is about 'thinking on one's feet'. Reflection-in-action is a very elusive and puzzling phenomenon. It is also difficult because care is dynamic and ever-changing. At each moment, something situation-specific is happening. More healthcare research is needed to understand it better.

Reflection-in-action generates a kind of knowledge on which we depend in order to perform our tasks spontaneously. It tells us something about the adequacy of our 'knowing-in-action' and it guides further action. Eraut (1995) looks at this in some detail and, in particular, at how reflection needs to be understood in relation to time (that is, when it occurs) and the context (the clinical situation in which we find ourselves) in which it occurs. In summary Eraut (1995) states that Schön's notion of reflection-in-action has at least three salient features.

1 Reflection being, at least in some measure, conscious, although it need not occur in one particular medium, such as in writing or in spoken words.
2 Reflection-in-action has a critical function, especially when asking the question: How has this current situation come to be this way?
3 Reflection gives rise to on-the-spot experiment as we respond to what is happening in front of us.

Reflection-on-practice (on-action)

This is Schön's second kind of reflection. It is usually taken to mean making sense of an action after it has occurred and learning something from the experience. What is learned may affect future action. It cannot affect the action being reflected upon because that has already passed. It is a way we come to know our 'tacit' knowledge. Reflection-on-practice can be practised individually or in team situations. It can be a private, solitary, introspective activity, or a more public, discursive, team-type. There are numerous ways to facilitate this kind of reflection, for example journal writing and critical incident analysis, using concept mapping, and role play, shared critical reading groups, story-telling, conversational analyses, visual art, poetry, music, combinations of all of these, and more. However, the distinction between reflection-in-action and reflection-on-practice may not be as clear as Schön and most subsequent writers imply. Eraut (1995) suggests that many practical processes can be construed as comprising several episodes, thus allowing them to be interpreted either as one single, but multi-phase action, or a series of successive but separate actions. So what might be considered reflection-in-action under the former interpretation becomes reflection-on-action under the latter interpretation. Eraut goes on to say that the preposition *on* should refer to the focus of reflection while the proposition *in* refers to the context of reflection. The alternatives to reflection-in-action are reflection before action, reflection after action and reflection away from or out of the action. Reflection-in-action and reflection-on-action are not dichotomous opposites.

Benefits of reflection - real or imagined?

It is right and proper to think carefully about the claims being made for reflective practice. Clarke *et al.* (1996) and Totterdell and Lambert (1999) offer some useful questions to bear in mind.

1 Can we say what this thing called 'reflective practice' is (can it be described or its impact felt)?
2 Can we specify when it happens (and under what conditions and within what time-frame)?
3 Can we be certain whether it can be taught/learned (and by whom) and what research evidence is there that it is effective?
4 Do we really know what it is for (is it, *inter alia*, a necessary condition for becoming a healthcare worker or a criterion for distinguishing professional from non-professional practice)?
5 Do we claim (or imply), or sound as if we claim, that reflective practice provides an epistemology for everyday clinical and professional healthcare practice?

The kinds of 'theoretical' knowledge we were describing earlier (universal, impersonal, general and objective), which downgraded practical knowledge, should not be rejected, rather it should no longer just be taken on trust. Postmodern thinking now asks such questions as: Who generates this knowledge? What power do they have? Who is being excluded as a consequence?

Being-human-well

This particular individualistic interest of reflection in 'being-human-well' is beautifully illustrated in two particular contributions by Chris Johns (Johns 2000b, 2001b). In 'Working with Alice: a reflection' (Johns 2000b) Chris sought to breathe life into the idea of reflection by writing a reflective journal and using a reflective lens, '. . . to become increasingly reflective within my practice, more sensitive to myself in relation to others, both patients and colleagues' (Johns 2000b, p. 203). In this article he shares 'the sacredness of the unfolding moment' with a patient called Alice, a woman with a terminal cancer. During his conversation with Alice, she mentions how much she enjoyed a foot massage. Chris spends 20 minutes working on both feet. He reflects, 'In my role as a nurse, when I place my hand on a person, I pause to tune myself into the other, to fuse our souls into a sacred healing dance. Being in tune with the other enhances the potential. It is most profound – beyond the scope of words . . . As nurses and therapists, we need to learn to be intentionally compassionate in non-attached ways so as to be available yet not take on board the distress and suffering of others as our own, otherwise we are at risk of becoming depleted and subsequently less available to the other. You will literally feel drained' (Johns 2000b, p. 201).

In 'The caring dance' (Johns 2001b) Chris again uses the 'being available' template as a frame to work holistically with patients and families. Through his meetings with Blackwolf and Gina Jones and his reading of Earth Dance Drum (Jones & Jones 1996) he invites us to consider the influence of Native American dance rituals. He says, 'So consider the caring dance as a ritual of being with another within a caring situation. Prepare for the caring dance, the dance of connection to yourself and to the patients and clients you work with' (Johns 2001b, p. 8).

An interest in being-human-well enables us to reflect upon the serious question: Which self is it that cares for patients? Our understanding of this can be enriched if we open our minds to the contributions from those from other fields and workplaces. For example, teachers in schools might ask themselves: Which self (me-as-teacher) is it that cares (teaches) for children (students)? There is a rich vein of reflective writing that can help us here (Loughran & Russell 2002, Samaras 2002). It is also useful to read the work of those particularly involved in the Self-Study of Teacher Education Practices (S-STEP). This is a special interest group (SIG) of the American Education Research Association. Their work is accessible from their website (www.ku.edu/~sstep).

The 'me' and the 'we': moving towards a team perspective

Four major social identity theories, two from sociology and two from psychology, act as more lenses through which to deepen our understanding of the practices of reflection. The first pair help develop our understandings of the me's (individualism), the latter pair the we's (teamness). Appealing to sociology first, briefly McCall and Simmons' (1978) role-identity theory incorporates both the 'I' and the 'me' aspects of the self. Role identity is a combination of the character and the role that individuals construct for themselves, as an occupant of a particular social and work position. The theory helps us appreciate that individuals carry out the broad expectations of their perceived social positions. This is the *role* part of role identity. It reflects the me. But they go on to explain how people do so with improvisations and presentations-of-self that make role performances expressive of personal character, idiosyncracies and 'quirks'. This is the *identity* part of role identity. In professional life we may only feel able to improvise and embellish the me's if our understanding of positions, roles and identities gives us room to do this, if they allow some latitude for creative, individualised or team performance. This is very relevant for any understanding of the way individuals behave in teams.

Second, Stryker's (1994) identity theory prepares us well for engaging with team learning and working presented later. Stryker's central interest was to try to explain why individuals choose to enact certain roles among the many available to them in their identity repertoires. For example, a person may hold the identities of doctor, father, Rotarian, friend, golfer, and so on, all of which collectively make up *him*-self. We may hold the identities of nurse, mother, churchgoer, footballer, painter, and so on, which all collectively make up the identities of *her*-self. We may hold combinations of identities of gay, chief executive, rebel, black, middle-class, divorcee, Protestant, able-bodied, and so on. Our identities refer to positions in (more or less) organised patterns of relationships, like teams, to which are attached sets of behavioural expectations and roles. So why do some people invest time and effort enacting certain roles rather than others? Why is it that a 'very nice person' becomes a monster when in the role of chairing a committee? Some of this can be explained by the notion of 'identity commitment'. We are committed to living out certain roles. A nurse may be committed to the role of mother or father. It is important to that nurse to be in the position of mother/father and playing that role. But to more fully understand this, in the context of this book, we need to link identity commitment to the notion of 'identity salience'.

The conception of salience I am using here refers to the likelihood that a person will enact a particular identity when given an opportunity to do so, or when avenues of possible action are felt to be open to them. Identity salience influences the actual enactment of social roles. The higher the salience of a particular identity, the more time and effort we may invest in its enactment. This begins a chaining of events, the more we attempt to perform well, the more one's self-esteem depends on that identity and the more one's identity performance reflects (general) shared values and norms. But we should also be interested in and perhaps be encouraging and supporting deviance. By this I mean deviating from and/or renegotiating the values and norms that we feel govern identity behaviour. This may actually liberate staff talents and applaud initiative. These are the 'I' aspects of self again, which are so important to know. The serious questions arising from all of this are:

1   How do I wish to construct my professional identity?
2   How do others affect this?
3   How do I continually negotiate my professional self?

The us and we's: a sense of team

In a relative sense there are much fewer published works, in healthcare, that link the practices of reflection with teams, than with groups, co-workers and individuals. What we do find are certain kinds of reflection used in groups and mainly in pre- and post-registration continuing professional development (CPD) contexts (Mountford & Rogers 1996, Platzer *et al.* 2000). Maybe Rolfe (2001) has a point when he says that reflective practices are merely, '... *a tool to be applied in order to meet the mandatory requirements for post-registration education*' (Rolfe 2001, p. 28). Often groups are organised into action learning sets (Haddock 1997). Sensibly I feel, Haddock does remind us that work in groups (and teams) brings with it certain risks. '*I contend that although a potentially ideal setting for learning, the group may evoke repressed anxiety and distress caused by self-awareness and contact with patients. This, if not contained, will hinder the process of learning from and through the experience. More rigorous attempts by those conducting such groups may be required, to maintain the boundary and thus the safety of the group, and to obtain supervision, in order to deal more effectively with problems arising'* (Haddock 1997, p. 381).

The practice of reflection with a focus on the 'us' has also been extensively discussed in the context of clinical supervision (Butterworth & Faugier 1997, Bishop 1998, Butterworth *et al.* 1998, Bond & Holland 1998, Ghaye & Lillyman 1998, Pritchard 1998). Historically there has been one dominant view of this process. It is one that is a particular expression of a supervisor-supervisee 'us-type' relationship. In my own work, and especially over the last five years from the work of my colleague Karen Deeny, we have come to celebrate a hybridity of views of clinical supervision. This is a consequence of asking staff what they want and need such a process to be like for them, in their own particular workplaces.

Through a partnership between the Institute of Reflective Practice and Worcestershire NHS (funded by a Workforce Development Confederation) and involving over 1500 health and social care staff, we have found that the principles and processes of inclusivity, of sharing learning, cultural literacy and of diversity within real and apparent similarity, to be a genuine basis for team learning and service improvement (see Part Four). The practice of reflection, where the 'we' is the team, is an emerging practice and policy imperative. There is also much to learn from work in other fields and outside health and social care. For example, Valkenburg & Dorst (1998) and Cossentino (2002) take Schön's original work forward as they explore the practices of reflection in the design studio.

Learning from another 'ology'

I am drawing selectively upon two theories from social psychology to enable us to understand more about teams. Specifically, I take a brief look at the important issue of collective identities. In Tajfel's (1981) social identity theory we find a definition of social identity as, '... *that part of an individual's self-concept which derives from his knowledge of his membership of a social group (or groups) together with the value and emotional significance attached to that membership*' (Tajfel 1981, p. 255). His theory is helpful because it shifts our attention away from individualism and to inter-*group* psychological processes. In his work he was particularly interested in understanding prejudice and social conflict, both relevant to effective team learning. Tajfel argued that what defined a group (or team in our case) was not its structure, function or size but the socially constructed reality of its members. This means that when individuals identify with a team, they begin to construct 'we' social identities (who we are), rather than 'me' social identities (who I am). Arguably, to nurture team-based healthcare cultures, staff need positive and distinctive team identities from which self-esteem and a sense of personal value can be derived. I pick this up again in Parts Three and Four. A serious question seems to be emerging, namely: How frequent and enduring are your experiences of 'we' compared with experiences of 'me' in your work? Clearly, our daily interactions may oscillate between the two, but my question to you is: Which is mostly true?

Turner *et al.*'s (1987) self-categorisation theory is also highly relevant to developing reflective teams. Their main interest was to understand collective behaviours. Whereas Tajfel's primary concern was with *intergroup* relations, especially group conflict and competition, Turner *et al.* focused attention on those processes that created a collective sense of self, which would make possible such phenomena as group cohesiveness, cooperation, altruism, emotional contagion and empathy, collective action, shared values and influencing processes. These are *intra-group* phenomena. What emerges from Turner *et al.*'s work is a question, namely: How do we shift from a personal to a collective identity? This takes us to a point about the importance of challenging the (alleged) cause-and-effect relations between collective identity and personal loss. In other words, that being part of a team (eg. a multi-professional team), with a particular identity, brings with it an inevitable loss of personal identity. Turner *et al.* described this as a process of depersonalisation. For example, they argued that group cohesiveness occurs when individuals perceive similarity between themselves and others in the group. It may be to do with similarities in thinking and practice. Group co-operation would occur because identifying oneself with others leads to a similarity of interests and goals. But depersonalisation can be problematic.

So how does all this enable us to extend our twin understandings of reflection as an interest in being-human-well and developing healthcare teams? Let me put it this way. What helps with a process like depersonalisation that Turner describes? Maybe at least four things. The first is to do with 'readiness'. We have to feel ready to join a particular team. This is a mix of past experiences, present expectations, values, ambitions and future options. The second is about 'fit'. By this I mean we may willingly become part of one particular team, rather than another, because we perceive fewer differences *among* us than *between* us and other staff. This of course makes a rather big assumption about what choices are actually open to us! The third is about 'desire'. This is about really wanting to be a part of the 'we'. This desire may arise from personal, professional and policy imperatives. The final influence is 'need', which may, for example, be due to the way we choose to express our contribution to care, and/or because of the local re-organisation of services and policy.

Inevitably these 'formal theories' (and there are many more) leave us with some unresolved questions about being-human-well and developing teams. For example, Tajfel and Turner *et al.* concentrate more on the cognitive than the emotional significance of the 'we'. Another issue is the blurring of the way social roles can be/are a basis for collective identities. There is much more to be said about the way certain identities serve different functions, in specific circumstances. For example, in the context of a 'long-hours' culture in the NHS and life/work balance initiatives, workaholics might become a new 'we'! Additionally 'over-workers' might become another kind of 'we' in spite of the risks we know from 'medical' knowledge (and other knowledges) about staff with these behaviours. If in the practice of reflection we keep the 'me' and 'we' as separate states, it is possible to raise some serious questions about the relationships between them. We need to understand better what triggers shifts from cultures of individualism ('I') towards collectivism ('we'). There can be difficulties with small, exclusive teams just as much as with large and highly inclusive ones.

Another important issue is how far cultures of individualism and collectivism can and should exist simultaneously. For example, in team working things like decision-making and cooperative action towards shared practices for patients, often require differentiated activities amongst team members. This specialisation and division of labour implies that various informal and formal roles are performed in the team. It is therefore possible to conceive that some members, say within a district nursing team, may be simultaneously aware of themselves as the one who goes to Professional Executive Committee meetings (role identity within the team) and as a team member working for the whole (collective identity) because of a large increase in the district nursing team's continence caseload. We know that we have multiple selves and identities (Ashmore & Jussim 1997). We know that people can see themselves in complex ways. Sometimes the 'me' as powerful, lively or awkward becomes a different 'me' when in the company of the 'we' (the team). Identities can be modified through enactment with other team members. But multiple identities can also be conjoined (e.g. clinical and activist) or fused within a single descriptive term (e.g. leader = older, experienced, authoritative). Such merged or fused identities may be somewhat resistant to change. Being-human-well suggests that we need to be concurrently aware of 'me' with 'we' and that this may modify the way each is enacted. This may well be a continuing and fertile area of interest for those practising reflection. The quality and pattern of relationships between team members can be described as the 'culture of care' within a team. I reflect on this in Part Four.

Chapter 7

An interest in embracing uncertainty: the practices of reflection as working with fuzziness and the challenges involved in service improvement and workplace transformation

I often hear people say, 'The only permanent thing in the NHS right now is change!' Behind this, for some, is a sense that much of the change consists merely of fads and fashions, hyped up by the latest gurus in the fields of practice development, human resource management, communications effectiveness, corporate cultures, one minute managers, TQMs, de-layering, downsizing, reengineering, balance scorecard advocates, and the like. Others say to me that working life is harder, less satisfying and more stressful. Some say that all they want to do is one thing well rather than a lot of things in a mediocre fashion. More tell me that they just wish the pace of change, reform and modernisation would slow down a bit, so that they feel they can 'get a grip on things'. These are expressions of change fatigue. What this implies is a desire to impose a pattern of meaning and stability upon their professional worlds. But what really needs to change? The world 'out there', only? Or maybe we need to engage in change ourselves? A change in the ways we see the world? The really good (team) leaders are those who enable members of the team to try to think and act differently, specifically through their willingness to change themselves rather than through trying to convince others that 'those others' are the only ones who need to change.

If the world of healthcare is perceived as one of instability, as a constant process 'surfing the white waters of change' and of uncertainty, then one natural response to this is to try to impose certainty upon it. For many this is equated with working even harder, faster, and longer hours. As a chair for the next Primary Care Trust locality managers meeting races in to the room I hear, '*Sorry everyone. I know I'm late. Just come from another meeting about NSF's for CHD and what CH(A)I are looking for. Can't stay long as I've got to get my head around the GMS stuff with HR people and the Q & O framework with GP's in N & S. And what's all this about worms and viruses? No don't answer that. Are we OK with MMR? We'll come to that. Right let's do away with the introductions and get down to business. Sorry but I've got to go by 3.45'.* As you listen to words issuing forth, many are ruing the fact that they left their NHS thesaurus behind! What a life! As most team leaders and NHS managers know, messengers bearing bad news are the first to be shot at. Yet if only good news is imparted when things are not going well, we get into real trouble.

Often for staff, much depends on the location of the driver for change and whether the team regards itself as a fashion-setter (innovatory in their practice with a team culture of innovation and influence) or fashion-takers (more reactive team cultures). What is apparent to me is the natural desire we have to try to make the complexity of modern service delivery and management more ordered, by sieving and sorting it in such a way that it becomes easier to understand. By doing this the worlds of work seem more tractable, more understandable, more meaningful. What I wish to highlight here is the increasing importance we need to attach to the 'management of meaning'.

Teams in the (fuzzy) zones

We live in an uncertain world. We cannot know everything. We make decisions based upon partial knowledge. The only thing that is certain is that nothing is certain. Because of this endemic uncertainty about the way we understand the world, our interactions and roles within it, we may have to make a choice. For example, on the one hand the world is both certain and knowable. This being the case, we go out to try to discover it, and the facts that exist. On the other hand we do not so much discover, as create, the worlds we inhabit through our own efforts. This is called a dualism or a binary opposite. Some other examples of binary opposites are black/white, win/lose, private/public, clean/dirty, self/other, appearance/reality, certainty/doubt, order/chaos (Peters 1989, Wheatley 1999). When we reduce the world to dualisms, we often do so because the world is too complicated to cope with otherwise. But doesn't this sound strange? Only to have two sides and that we have to choose which side we are on? That we are either in or out of a team. We are one of them or they are one of us? That one side is telling the truth or they are not? Perhaps we need to reassure ourselves that we can include continua in the way we describe who we are, what we do and with whom? In other words the world is a lot more 'fuzzy' and uncertain than I am suggesting. We are not just happy or sad but 'chilled out'. We are not busy or bored but working at a steady pace. Not leading or following but alongside.

Being a competent professional brings with it an awareness of where the divisions lie in our professional worlds. Sometimes these divisions (dualities) are not really out there, we just think they are. Sometimes we impose this or that particular division on the world and so turn complexity into something more understandable. Our mindset should be an open one. As mentioned earlier, open-mindedness was one of three attributes that Dewey (1933) suggested were essential for reflective practitioners. By open-mindedness he meant being aware of our prejudices and biases, partisanship and other dispositions that serve to close the mind and make it unwilling to entertain new ideas. This relates to the team's ability to 'think differently'.

A sense of certainty

One of the key factors in shaping an attitude of openness is how we individually and collectively (in teams) perceive certainty. '*A sense of who we are and what we stand for is essential to our mental health. We all need anchor points of some sort to help us retain a grip on reality. If our sense of certainty is undermined, the way we think shifts. In order to be able to work smarter rather than harder as a reflex reaction to change, we need to understand and manage our perceptions about certainty*' (Reid 2002, p. 67). How far do we need a sense of certainty? This varies between individuals and teams and over time. Also the nature of what we need to be certain about in our healthcare work will vary. A sense of certainty will also depend upon the confidence we have in ourselves and in our relationships with others in our team. The rhetoric of practising reflection is that the old certainties of tradition, custom, technical efficiency and so on are rejected (Schön 1983, 1987, 1992). The new certainty is that everything is open-to-doubt (Parker 1997), to scrutiny and question, this includes the established 'truths' and the ways of doing things around which practice is anchored. 'The capacity to articulate doubt becomes the mark of the attitude of seriousness... this idea of open-mindedness, the exhortation *constantly* to question, criticise and change, issues in a culture of *radical doubt*' (Parker 1997, p. 122) (Parker's italics). The world is fuzzy. We practise without certainty. We provide healthcare in an uncertain world (Mullavey-O'Byrne & West 2001). We might therefore energetically consider ways of making this fuzziness more understandable and less threatening. There is much work that demonstrates this interest in embracing uncertainty.

Fuzzy worlds and action-driven healthcare professionals

There is a great deal of interest in the practices of reflection that depict ways to *learn through*. For example, we learn through critical or significant incident analysis, through concept mapping, journals, stories, and so on. All of these are purported to be methods used in the spirit of reflecting on practice, that help us make sense of ourselves, our practices and the contexts in which they are embedded. They try to bring some added clarity to our fuzzy worlds. In the language of chaos theory (Gleick 1991) these methods help us create a kind of 'bounded disorder'. Everything is not certain or uncertain (another dualism) but both and shades in-between. The critical thing is knowing the difference. This mindset, for me anyway, is much more appropriate to twenty-first century NHS working life. The modern manager for a modern NHS and the modern team (which I will propose later is a reflective one) are able to work creatively and competently at the fuzzy margins of order and chaos in service delivery systems.

The background and development of learning through reflections on 'critical incidents' can be traced to Flannagan (1954). It has been seen as a useful approach to making sense of 'fuzziness' in nursing practice (Clamp 1980, Minghella & Benson 1995, Parker *et al.* 1995, Rich & Parker 1995, Love 1996, Chesney 1996, Ghaye & Lillyman 1997) and in education through the work of Tripp (1993). He defines such incidents thus, 'Incidents happen, but critical incidents are produced by the way we look at a situation, it is an interpretation of the significance of an event' (Tripp 1993, p. 8). From nursing, for example, we find one way to present it thus, '*Snapshot views of the daily work of the nurse and by examining them, the effects of care on patients can be seen and interactions between colleagues can be highlighted*' (Clamp 1980, p. 1756). In healthcare the 'criticality' of an incident is value-laden and the word can be ambiguous. Some prefer to refer to these incidents as moments of 'significant learning'. I suggest that a key characteristic is that these should be incidents *from* practice, not *about* practice. By this I mean the person/team needs to have an actual attachment to the incident. It might be about them and their work in their clinical area. An incident about practice may be useful, illuminative and even worth reflecting upon. But it may well lack 'criticality' in the sense that the genesis of the incident is not from the individual's/team's own working life.

Making practice visible

Sometimes in our pursuit to try to make practice more understandable, we have to make it more visible to ourselves. In other words we have to externalise our thinking. We have to portray some of it in such a way that it becomes possible to look at it, ask questions about it and check it out. One practical way this can be done is through a method called mind mapping or concept mapping (Daley 1996, Caelli 1998). I have found this to be very helpful in some situations of enhancing team learning (Ghaye & Lillyman 2000). Briefly, a concept map is a special type of picture containing different kinds of information. This information is arranged in a way so that relationships can be seen and understood by the 'map readers'. The information is spatially organised. The fundamental elements are:

1 *Nodes*. These are the key ideas (concepts) which the team have agreed will be the catalyst for reflection.
2 *Links*. These are the lines members draw between the nodes. They do not have to be straight ones but do symbolise some link or meaning, in the team member's mind, between two or more of the ideas.

3   *Labels*. These are the words that staff write on their links to express
    what they feel are the connections between two or more nodes. More
    than one link may connect two nodes.

Constructing reality maps

What emerges are personal and collective 'reality' maps. Usually everyone's map is different. Members can make a map. They might then be
invited to compare maps in pairs, fours and so on until a team picture is
built up. It does not have to be limited to an A4-sized paper exercise.
I have found that big can be better, in other words an invitation to build
large maps on the table and/or floor, moving pieces of paper around and
connecting them up with strips of coloured card. All the time staff need to
be talking to each other about their thinking with regard to one or more
of the ideas being explored. An interesting variant on the map is a
'line' (Orland 2000). This is where team members are invited to draw
freely a line, or lines, of any length and shape, that they feel constitutes
significant felt experiences. Members are then asked either to write or to
talk through the significance of the representation. This is a further
example of how we might broaden the bandwidth of activities we
use to try to embrace a fuzzy world. Like maps, the line provides
us with an opportunity for elucidating tacit aspects of our personal and
professional knowledge. Orland (2000, p. 197) argues, 'In particular, its
application seems especially relevant for . . . agendas that focus on participant's perceptions of complex, dynamic and personally 'charged' experiences . . .'.

Research in cognitive psychology has been marked by a proliferation of
ways to represent information stored in our memory. Some early discussions and representations that are helpful to consult are Aitkenhead &
Slack (1993), Johnson (1969), Mayer (1970), Scott (1966) and Shavelson
(1974). Much more recently, and in healthcare are Burns & Grove (1993)
and Irvine (1995). A very comprehensive text about the educative potency of this approach, which is essentially about creating and using
knowledge to enable us to learn better, is Novak (1998).

Getting team learning into the open

Figures 7.1 and 7.2 show individual maps from a newly formed intermediate care team of 32 members. Using a snowballing process, initial
groups of four staff made their own 'map' and then incorporated it with
others. This was a constant process of re-construction and team meaning-
making. It took staff 45 minutes to build the two maps shown. After
making these maps staff were invited to:

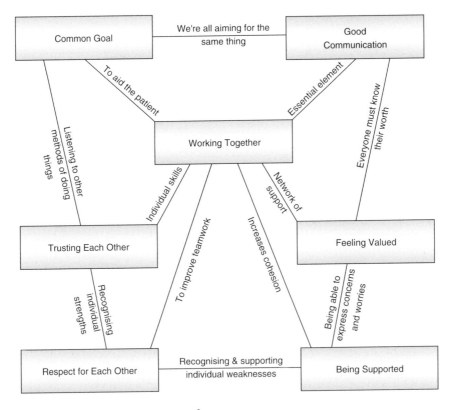

Fig 7.1 Getting learning into the open.

- Look for similarities and differences between the two maps.
- Spend some time exploring and explaining.

The spatial arrangement of each map tells us something quite signifi-cant about how staff 'see' things. Staff need to share their thoughts about which idea they placed on their paper first, and why. Which second and why. Sometimes the map tells a kind of linear story. This is a chaining of ideas. One idea (node) is put down first, which leads to the next and so on until there is a continuous 'big think' expressed on the page. Sometimes a map might show the centrality of a 'big idea' for a team and how other ideas add more meaning and are supportive of it. What is more signifi-cant is the nature of the links between the nodes. Staff should be encour-aged to add more significant nodes if they wish. Maps can vary in their complexity of form and content. If the same ideas are used, a mapping activity done at a later date can be compared with an earlier map. What I am saying here is that we need to find ways to enable teams to *talk to learn*. These cannot normally be elaborate and costly but activities that can be done relatively quickly and cheaply. If the activity can be both practical and 'fun' then so much the better. But we should remember, all learning is not always fun.

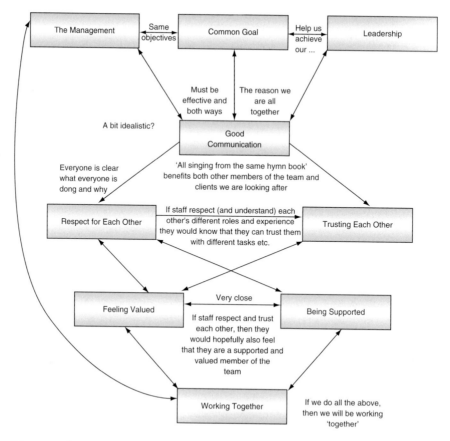

Fig 7.2   Concept mapping.

In the process of developing teams, staff need to be open to ideas from everywhere. It is unwise for us to think that we have all the answers to making 'our' fuzziness more understandable. One characteristic of the reflective team is that they never stop trying to search out new ideas. They always try to be open and receptive to ideas from everywhere. They certainly let each other in the team know that they want to hear from them. They celebrate when a member comes up with a good idea. New ideas do not intimidate team members. Ideas energise them. Even better is when ideas are then acted upon. This tends to motivate others to express their ideas as well. When we think we know it all, we stop learning! Learning to understand the fuzziness of practice that arises from these uncertainties is essential: '... feeling unsure, realising that our actions sometimes contradict our words, or admitting that we are not in control of every event in our practice are anathema to many of us. We believe that unless we anticipate every eventuality and respond appropriately, we are failing. Appearing confused, hesitant, or baffled seems a sign of weakness. And admitting that we feel tired, unmotivated, or bored seems a betrayal of the humanitarian zest we are supposed to exhibit' (Brookfield 1990, p. 3).

Storying that embraces fuzziness

Storying might be a helpful practice of reflection for teams. My reason for saying this is the current focus by government, NHS agencies and trusts on 'the patient's journey' and 'the discovery interview'. In addition to confessional writing, this takes us into narrative knowing through bio-graphical, autobiographical, psycho-biographical and even 'detective' genres. I want to link this to the development of teams as it helps us understand the serious question: How far does good team working and learning translate into a good service? Learning from service user stories is one way we might be able to become clearer about this question. But first, four points about trying to embrace fuzziness through storying.

1   When team members tell or create stories it is an acknowledgement that they know something (but not everything) of the issue from the inside.
2   If team members choose to learn through storying there needs to come a time when they ask themselves, 'What has made this a good story for us?'
3   If a team finds itself locked into habitual practices and symbolic routines, where the busyness of working life dulls and makes us blind to that which is 'special', which is personally regenerating and collectively re-affirming, then there may be no surprises, no good ideas and exchanges. In other words there may be no stories to tell (Rosenfeld & Tardieu 2000).
4   *Storying can be seen as a practice of reflection that might bring some new understandings and help us embrace fuzziness. 'Sense is crafted, put together with skill and care, not simply experienced as if prefabricated. We can see others, and occasionally ourselves, making sense in a way which does not seem to be conductive to productive action; it is not simply that sense is made or not made, but that there are consequences to the kind of sense that is made. Everyday sense-making is not a matter of trying to make total sense of everything. There are levels of sense with which we feel comfortable. Too much sense – too clear an understanding of everything around us – may be boring'* (Wallemaq & Sims 1998, p. 121).

In the context of the individual (team member, patient) and the collect-ive (the whole team) it is important to try to look at an emerging story in different ways so that we can see, hear and try to understand the com-plexities and richness of it (Coffey & Atkinson 1996). We need to reflect upon the 'whys' (why the story is being told), the 'hows' (how it is being told) the 'whats' (what is being included, the story's content) and the 'what nots' (what is not being re-told, why and how we might know or sense this). Making sense of a story is linked to coherence. We often understand something better if it 'hangs together' in some meaningful way. But '... the notion of coherence in the telling of life histories is a contested issue' (Smith & Sparkes 2002, p. 144). Smith and Sparkes go on to report the work of Holstein and Gubrium (2000) when they say, '... *while experience can provide an endless supply of potentially reportable storyable items; it is the incorporation of particular items into a coherent account that gives them meaning. Thus storytelling is an ongoing process of composition. Stories do not come fully formed or organised on their own ... there is a persistent interplay between what is available for conveying a story and how a particular narrative unfolds in practice; it is from this interplay that both self-coherence and diversity develop*' (Smith & Sparkes 2002, p. 144–45).

Stories are potentially full of tensions and contradictions, things said, half-told and left unsaid. The complexities in each story are unique and perhaps we should try to preserve this. Some have argued that we have a natural desire to tell stories, '... *that humans are storytelling creatures who, individually and socially, lead storied lives and tell stories of those lives*' (Clandinin & Connelly 1995, p. 154). This act of storytelling is a relational act because stories are often told to others. There is a reciprocity in the telling and in the responding. Additionally '... *storying is a reflective act. Stories are not icons to be learned but inquiries on which further inquiry takes place through their telling and through response to them*' (Clandinin & Connelly 1995, p. 156).

Of course, wanting to tell and write 'good' team stories is not the same as saying we want to hear 'successful' ones. From a patient's perspective in, '... *wanting to hear stories about "recovery", we may not only be complicit in sustaining and reproducing culturally preferred stories that might be disempowering, but we may also interfere with people's rights to tell their own tales, tales that may lack the coherence, plot, or resolution we, and they, desire*' (Smith & Sparkes 2002, p. 167). Narratives, and stories in particular, that team members tell each other, are very important because they provide an opportunity to understand something of the fuzziness of our practice worlds. '*We live in a sea of stories, and like the fish who (according to the proverb) will be the last to discover water, we have our own difficulties grasping what it is like to swim in stories. It is not that we lack competence in creating our narrative accounts of reality, far from it. We are, if anything, too expert. Our problem, rather, is achieving consciousness of what we so easily do automatically*' (Bruner 1996, p. 147).

Reflection and its interest in chaos

Chaos theory reminds us that patterns actually exist where and when we thought the 'world' was random, formless and spontaneous. Chaos is not just complicated, pattern-less action. It is more subtle than this. Stewart (1989, 1995) and Stewart and Golubitsky (1992) argue that chaos is 'apparently' complicated, 'apparently' pattern-less behaviour. If we can be creative in the reflective lenses used to see, then patterns and hidden rhythms in the fuzziness of practice may become discernible. Reflective practices with an interest in embracing uncertainty help us ask certain questions about the patterns we observe. Questions to do with how and why the patterns in practice exist, where they have come from, how we might influence and shape them and what practical use we might make of what we have learned through appreciating patterns in our work. We should not forget that we live in a universe of patterns. *'Every night the stars move in circles across the sky. The seasons cycle at yearly intervals. No two snowflakes are ever exactly the same, but they all have a six-fold symmetry. Tigers and zebras are covered in patterns of stripes, leopards and hyenas are covered in patterns of spots. Intricate trains of waves march across the oceans; very similar trains of sand dunes march across the desert. Coloured arcs of light adorn the sky in the form of rainbows, and a bright circular halo sometimes surrounds the moon on winter nights ... Patterns possess utility as well as beauty. Once we have learned to recognise a background pattern, exceptions suddenly stand out. The desert stands still but the lion moves'* (Stewart 1995, pp. 1–3).

Reflection and symmetry

There is something attractive about symmetry. Perhaps it is its repetitive-ness and therefore predictability that attracts us. Cognitively and aesthet-ically some find symmetry appealing. Maybe it is its association with 'mirror images'. There are parallels here between this and aspects of clinical practice. Some health care professionals welcome and actively seek the appeal of *practice-as-symmetry*. We have repetitive routines and predictable patterns of work. We can wrap ourselves up in these. They often become what is called our 'taken-for-granted' clinical worlds. They can act as a comfort blanket offering a sense of security that comes from knowing what is likely to come and be needed next. There are many kinds of symmetry. Some of the most important kinds are *flips, turns* and *slides*. For example, we often talk about 'flipping things over' to try to understand the practice phenomenon another way. We flip things over in order see 'the other side of things'. Rotation or 'turning' is that kind of symmetry which is to do with rotating objects around a fixed point, like a wheel turning around its hub. It is about rotating objects through different angles about the same axis. In using reflection to help us understand fuzziness we need to 'turn things around' and actively consider a variety of other points of view on the same issue.

Sliding is a particular type of symmetry where transformations occur when an object or objects are slid along without rotating them. Slides can incorporate both horizontal and vertical movements. An array of bath-room tiles, the bees' honeycomb, are examples of this kind of symmetry, where the 'tiles' are repeated and can be moved around in the construc-tion process. Again, this kind of thinking is useful and can be employed to make sense of our clinical practice. It is useful to 'move things around' a bit like the pieces of a jigsaw. As we slide one piece of practice we not only align it with another but we create a space behind it for new insights, for further pieces of the puzzle to move into. All this repositioning creates new pictures of practice. It is all done within a fixed frame too. The 'image' is bounded. This edge might be the ward, unit or department, within which we work. It might be bounded by a National Service Framework, and so on.

Breaking symmetry is another process that may enable us to work creatively in our fuzzy worlds. Broken symmetry occurs when the existing patterns are disturbed. Something has to bring this about, to 'trigger' it. I will be suggesting later that the practice of reflection as asking serious questions, is just such a trigger. Resistance is an excellent example where the symmetries of practice break reluctantly. It is important to remember that as teams endeavour to improve their thinking and actions, some symmetries of practice *have* to be broken. The point is that when we break an existing symmetry of practice rather a lot of it often survives. It is still present, in the 'system'. It is there in another form or exists in another way. Memories of 'what things were like', feelings about 'how things were around here', 'old habits dying hard' and ways of working that cannot be easily un-learned are examples of fragments of former symmetries of practice.

Chapter 8

An interest in the bottom line: the practices of reflection as improving practice and getting results

I recently attended a one-day conference called 'accelerating productivity and quality'. It was essentially a day for those who wanted to reflect upon the ways teams of 'modern managers and modern management processes' might help improve health and social care services. The sub-text for the day was all about the 'bottom line'. Two views of this tended to permeate discussions. First, a view of trying to identify the key, crucial and deciding factors and influences that would improve services and how far these could be measured. Second, a view of the bottom line, for individual services and organisations, as what they wanted, ultimately to achieve. It was results, targets and outcomes focused. We now know that 'if we always do what we've always done, we will always get what we've always got!' For some this is a great trigger for thinking and acting differently. Another homily is that 'if you don't know where you are going, any road will do'. Because the intention of the day was explicitly 'improving healthcare productivity and quality' it fell comfortably in the arena of (collective) reflection as trying to make something better.

Getting behind the bottom line

At the conference the bottom line was addressed (or alluded to) by much talk about 'value streams', 'lean thinking', 'balancing scorecards', 'benchmarking', 'financial flows', and so on. Over coffee and lunch the talk shifted to 'making things better' in 'neurotic organisations' and challenging 'Mintzberg-type configurations'. What a day! So what did I learn? First, that the practices of reflection can help teams understand how things impact on their bottom line and particularly within 'doing more with less' cultures. Second, that teams can draw upon the practices of reflection to open up their thinking (and therefore possibilities for acting differently) by considering multiple bottom lines. Arguably we are moving into a 'triple bottom line' culture in the NHS linked to economics (resourcing services), social interactions (staff with patients and the public) and environment (the sites where services are accessed). Third, the practices of reflection can enable teams to move from bottom-line to more top-line thinking and actions. By this I mean lifting our heads up a little more to see where the horizons are and to try to see the roads ahead more clearly. One consequence of rapid change is that it tends to force us to 'get our heads down' at the very time when we should be doing the opposite! Fourth, much more work needs to be done with planning teams to enable them to get behind the bottom line. Business excellence models in the NHS are dominated by finance, power, strategies, partnering, ambition, innovation, stewardship and the like. The practices of reflection might enable us to consider how this might be helpfully infused by 'spiritual wisdom' (Graves & Addington 2002, Ghaye 2005), knowledge of soul-friendly businesses (Lamont 2002) and how we might take our soul to work and not just our business plans (Peppers & Briskin 2000).

. Finally, I re-learned that we need to be cautious of linear thinking, in any direction. For example, we do not magically turn dysfunctional, troubled, poorly performing teams into successful ones. We do not move from bottom to top-line thinking without a struggle. There is more than one trajectory (Miller 1990). More than one route that teams can take and it is not always towards improving their working lives or being in a better world! When the heat is on, with targets that need to be met, and the system is under pressure, there are some trajectories that lead, unfortunately, from success to failure. I caricature thus:

- *The focusing trajectory.* Where teams of highly skilled, experienced professionals and support staff, committed to quality service provision, scientists and artists, true 'crafts' women and men, turn into rigidly controlled, detail-obsessed, target-frenzied tinkerers.
- *The venturing trajectory.* Where imaginative team leaders working together with staff to build innovative, influential boundary-crossing teams, turn into greedy and grabbing imperialists, guarding resources and turf jealously, not daring to venture into the world of (apparent) chaos, where opportunities abound, anymore.
- *The inventing trajectory.* Where teams that nurture a culture of questioning, that are accepting ideas from everywhere, which thrive on diversity, turn into utopian escapists who are accused of losing the plot, airy-fairy thinking, theorists speaking psycho-babble.
- *The decoupling trajectory.* Where teams that take partnership and participation seriously, that cleverly add value to what they can do for patients by working with others, turn into escape committee chair persons, protecting their backs, who retreat into boxes because that is the last place left to them where they feel some sense of security and personal worth.

Through the practices of reflection we can, at least, come to know the nature of being 'trapped' in one (or more) of these trajectories and perhaps better understand that teams have a shelf-life. They come and go, and are more or less successful.

Reflection on energy, not time management

The time management movement of the 1980s and 1990s helped some staff become more productive. But at what cost? Time is finite. There are only 24 hours in a day. Having reflected upon the accumulated human cost to some staff in terms of increasing stress, burnout, sickness rates, depression, prolonged multi-tasking, broken marriages, and so on, managing energy has become more important than managing time. Energy is a team's most precious resource. It is the basic currency of performance. Using it is how a team achieves results. Most of the qualities team members need to do their job confidently and compassionately require energy in abundance. We need to reflect upon how teams can build and sustain their energy levels. High performing healthcare teams are not simply physically energised, but also emotionally connected, mentally focused and spiritually aligned with values and actions bigger than staff's individual self-interests. Loehr and Swartz (2005) elaborate upon the notion of energy. They state that physical energy is about the *quantity* of it. At the emotional level it is more to do with its *quality*. Often we describe this as positive or negative energy. At a mental level it is the *focus* of our energy that is crucial. Getting and staying focused is crucial to getting results. Finally, at the spiritual level it is the *force* of energy in teams that helps them get results. It is about the energy of the human spirit. A powerful source of this is when staff are able to align their values with those of the organisation.

Goleman's (1997) work on emotional intelligence and capacity, Seligman's (2004) work on managing our cognitive capacity, and Covey (1999) are texts which elucidate the spiritual dimension of everyday effectiveness. They are becoming 'must' reads for twenty-first century reflective teams. So this interest of the practices of reflection in the bottom line, is bringing with it an interest in being 'fully engaged'. For healthcare teams I suggest this requires us to systematically reflect upon three fundamental aspects of achieving results.

1   Those aspects of working life that deplete and restore a team's energy levels.
2   How teams renew themselves emotionally, mentally and spiritually, not just physically. What these practices and rituals are.
3   How teams might 'strategically disengage'. By this I mean reflecting on what members say about stress and recovery and their views on 'work-rest' ratios. Teams need to reflect seriously on the ways they might look at their energy expenditure against their energy recovery. Simply using measures of how relentlessly staff push themselves is madness. We need to change the value set and the cultures in some NHS workplaces so that rest and recovery are not regarded as signs of weakness and inefficiency. Full engagement requires periodic disengagement. This does not mean having a coffee break and continuing

to talk about pressing work issues. We have to get off the current 'thinking track'. The quality of a team's recovery time is crucial. It is when real healing, regeneration and renewal takes place. If teams do not reflect on these issues they are likely to become energy bankrupt. Of course there is another scenario. Too much recovery without sufficient energy expenditure can lead to atrophy, boredom and dis-enchantment.

Heath and Freshwater (2000) say we should avoid 'inappropriate in-tent'. It goes back to what I said earlier (see Orientation). There are no silver bullet cures to 'making something better'. We are urged to think carefully about the nature of reflection (Kinsella 2001, Rodgers 2002) and what reflecting in and on action means (Clinton 1998). We are encour-aged not to be fashion victims (Hulatt 1995, Hagland 1998) and that we should consider its strengths and weaknesses carefully (Hannigan 2001). There are interesting and important arguments that see reflection as a flawed strategy for the nursing profession (Mackintosh 1998) and that it is a necessary, but not a sufficient condition for professional development (Day 1993). This, I believe, provides a glimpse of a healthy and lively dialogue. I do not necessarily see this as symptomatic of practices that have lost their way. Something I have learned in building reflective teams is that they practice with 'mind wide open'. Maybe we need to keep learning about how to move in this world unaided by certainty? Losing a little helps in finding a little. Perhaps we need to lose our obsession with answers and focus more on the importance of asking questions first.

Chapter 9

An interest in reflection as the art of asking serious questions

Does this sound a bit destabilising? A bit negative? In general the point here is that we can view this particular interest as a further kind of practice. It is about a team being involved in thinking critically and creatively in order to ask certain kinds of question. This involves a preparedness to challenge customary understandings. Seriousness is reflected in a team's ability to articulate doubt. I wonder what you normally do when you don't know what to do? What do you do when you make a mistake or when you appreciate that you might have done something better by doing it differently? How often do you submit yourself to a process of self-flagellating guilt? Maybe it is more self-delusional denial? How often do you weigh yourself down and beat yourself up with feelings of failure? Maybe it is more a case of trying to deny that anything much is wrong or inappropriate? Put rather negatively, there are risks in asking serious questions, For example:

- burning ourselves out;
- crucifying ourselves on the cross of perfection;
- fruitless martyrdom;
- falling victim to a feeling that we are not making any kind of difference to the lives of those we work with and care for; and
- being consumed by pessimism about the limits of our own influence to genuinely make a difference to the quality of patient care.

Teams need to pay attention to their own survival. This is not narcissistic conceit but a fundamental and proper thing to do, especially in times of rapid NHS modernisation. To do this I suggest they need to know what constitutes the 'serious questions' that need to be asked (and responded to) to achieve this. For team leaders and managers they may need to learn to let go of a desire to fully control change, thus leaving more room for the team to self-organise. A crucial point of entry into real (and perceived) chaos is when team leaders and managers take the decision *not* to try to 'control' the process anymore, but instead to allow teams to work out, for themselves, what constitutes safe, ethical and legal practice in a changing workplace, and appropriate clinical standards, with regard to local circumstances and case loads.

With lots of this-and-that s, maybe s, and what if s, all soaking up a lot of energy, the key is to know when to let go and when to intervene. We all too readily commit to the belief that events can be controlled and when we find that this is difficult or impossible, we are presented with a mental

dilemma. Psychologists call this 'cognitive dissonance'. It is those moments when things do not happen the way we say, or hoped, they would.
Often we invest much personal and collective effort in the belief that we
can 'make things happen', and when this eludes us, our self and collective esteem can suffer. This often causes defence mechanisms to kick in.
We use these to protect ourselves. Our good plans and intentions may
then become a target of sabotage-by-others. We never consider that these
'others' may indeed be us! Blame becomes a hot topic of conversation. We
forget our history together. Our futures disappear. Letting go is anathema to some. Perhaps we need to learn to let go and see where this leads
us.

Schön's 'serious' questions

In his classic book *The Reflective Turn* (Schön 1991, p. 5) poses a number of
serious questions that attempt to 'give practitioners reason', particularly
when practice appears to be strange or puzzling. The answers to these
questions are encapsulated by a process of '... reflection on the understandings already built into the skilful actions of everyday practice'
(Schön 1991, p. 5). Thus practitioner's '... primary concern is to discover... *what they already understand and know how to do'*. Beguilingly
simple perhaps? Some of his questions are:

1   What do practitioners need to know?
2   What is it appropriate to reflect upon?
3   What is an appropriate way of observing and reflecting on practice?
4   When we have taken the reflective turn, what constitutes appropriate
    rigour?

   What Schön is getting at here is that professional life is a matter of
learning from and responding appropriately to events and situations as
they are experienced. This is about being adept. It is also linked to the
performative discourse where competence resides in the humanistic
discourse of reflection as self-development and self-empowerment. Barnett (1997, p. 132) says that Schön is telling us nothing new. He argues
that, '... *professionals simply are reflective practitioners; that is partly what we
mean by the term professional'*. Professional life in the NHS is promoting
more team-based learning and working. A culture of teamness where
peer judgement and the sense of worth and identity that comes from peer
connectedness do not sit easily with the notion of the individual practitioner.
   For some, the practice of reflection brings with it a commitment to
'dare to be political', to overcome constraints that cause us to accept
extant power structures. Some argue that a political dimension in Schön's
work is 'totally missing' (Smyth 1991, p. 107). Additionally, reflection
occurs in a social context. There is a worrying aspect to Schön's work

which seems to under-state this. Smyth (1991, p. 107) expresses it thus, *'What is missing from his conceptualisation is any acknowledgement of the socially constructed nature of knowledge. His notion of the reflective appears to remain trapped within a psychologistic framework that regards knowledge as being acquired solely through the systematic application of cognitive skills to particular situations'.*

What are the qualities of a serious question?

The word 'serious' has many connotations. A condition or incident may be seriously life-threatening. Being over-spent and running into debt, may be a serious thing for us. Not achieving the star rating we wanted and losing good staff, may be regarded as serious also. We can speak seriously, make a serious point or, as we 'get down to the wire', we may hear ourselves say, 'Now things are really becoming serious'. And what about questions? Sometimes questions are known, defined and asked by us, sometimes for us. On other occasions questions are responded to by us, sometimes on our behalf. I offer a particular collection of qualities that characterise a serious question. A serious question is:

1   *Our question.* Serious questions are someone's questions. They are our questions. By this I mean that the question concerns the team, the us and the we I discussed earlier. If it is a question about practice and clinical action, then it is *our* practice. It is the work we are involved in or with. They are serious because they are about what we did, are doing, or hope to do. They are therefore about successes, doubts, decisions and actions. *Our* decisions and how they might affect us and those we work with and care for. The team not only frames and poses the question, but through responding to it, call themselves in to question. The team has to account for itself. What influences the nature of the question might be some aspect of practice or policy from 'elsewhere' (outside the team) or from within. The essential point is that, whatever its source, the team is or becomes involved with it. The team owns the questions.

2   *Value-laden.* Serious questions are predicated upon a team first being able to articulate 'This is what we stand for'. The seriousness of the question is linked to their desire to live more fully their values in their practice. I make no claim here that what might be regarded as a serious question for one team, may be regarded in a similar way by others. They emanate from the team's successes, felt concerns or sense of unease and their commitment to be true to themselves. Because of their connections with the team's values, everyone has an interest in and commitment to them. The value/s that the question/s connect with give the team good reasons for asking them. Serious questions

can therefore be asked in cases where we are being called upon to justify our practices. For example, they can be used to question:

- tradition (how things have always been done);
- bias (how I like it to be done);
- dogma (this is the 'right' way to do it); and
- ideology (as required by the current orthodoxies).

These are serious because they question both ends and means in healthcare.

3 *Ethically situated.* Serious questions are ethical ones and situated. Ethics is central to healthcare. For some it is associated with 'big dilemmas' (Simons & Usher 2000; Quallington 2000). In the Nursing and Midwifery Council's Code of Professional Conduct (2002) it states in clause 8.1 '*As a registered nurse, midwife or health visitor, you must act to identify and minimise the risks to patients and clients ... you must work with other members of the team to promote healthcare environments that are conducive to safe, therapeutic and ethical practice*' (NMC 2002, p. 9). So not only are serious questions particular to a given team but also to a point in time and with regard to a particular service. In other words they are situated. An ethically situated question is mediated by the local and specific. It is also situated culturally and historically.

4 *Imbued with a sense of criticality.* Criticality is an expression of political engagement. In asking serious questions the team is conscious of the fact that they are engaging in a political act. For example, an interest in the bottom line and making something better, is a political act. It involves both understandings and actions with regard to who gets what, where, how and why. Questioning in this way also demonstrates the team's ability to reflect on its own assumptions and practices as people of a particular cultural and historical formation. It demonstrates that the team's values are perpetually open to challenge because of the effects that actioning these values have upon others. Criticality is a function of the teams collective questioning. It is therefore always social in character. This sense of criticality might involve questioning the evidence base of something, or questioning the motivation behind why the team or service user group act in the way they do. Asking serious questions is using a *language of critique.*

5 *Impregnated with power.* Power is everywhere, not because it is all-embracing, but because it comes from everywhere. Power circulates within a team. So it would be wise not to separate power from knowledge. Within each team there is a plurality of power and knowledge relations, which are exercised by staff during different aspects of their work, for example in regular team meetings, team briefs, clinical practice, and so on. A serious question problematises the interplay between power and knowledge. This at least gives the team the opportunity to 'free themselves from themselves'. Because

serious questions are impregnated with power they provide us with the opportunity to look again at how we conduct ourselves, professionally with patients, in accordance with a duty of care, codes of conduct and the Hippocratic Oath. Teams are not power-free zones!

6   *Associated with creative space.* A question's seriousness is reflected by the way it constructively challenges a team's 'limits'. This refers to customary forms of thought and action. In other words that which is taken for granted, something explicitly claimed and acknowledged as a limit to thinking and acting. Asking these kinds of questions, in team-based work cultures, can open up a space to be devoted to the creative act of trying to think and act differently. This is close to Freire's (1972) view that thinking fuels action and vice versa. He argued that criticality required both reflection and action, interpretation and change. '*Critical consciousness is brought about not through intellectual effort alone but through praxis – through the authentic union of action and reflection*' (Freire 1972, p. 48). Space in which to be creative is dependent upon the nature of team cultures, which I present in some detail in Part Four. In creative spaces we can engage in a *language of possibility*. Here team members are open to hear things differently. They size up the world differently. They step outside customary frames of reference. It is not a serious question if it can be adequately addressed and dealt with from within the framework of customary mindsets and behaviours.

7   *Have to be asked.* Serious questions are those that the team believe have to be asked. They are moving questions. Their seriousness moves us to do something. Their nature makes us impassioned to pursue them rigorously. When a team regards its practice as being troublesome, puzzling or difficult and in need of improvement, matters become serious and serious questions have to be asked. But when practice is highly successful, fulfilling and publicly acknowledged, serious questions often dry up. Serious questions can be asked in times of deficit and difficulty but need to be asked in times of joy and celebration. Seriousness can kick in at some quite unexpected moments. A chance encounter with a colleague, a comment made by a patient, an e-mail from a manager asking you to attend a meeting, an unexpected shortfall in bed availability, staff or revenue. Serious questions are also timely ones. 'It's right that we ask this now.' They seize the moment. 'Say it now, don't let's ponder on it endlessly.' 'That was the opening you'd been waiting for to ask the question.' It is not only readiness and alertness to the unfolding moment that characterises its seriousness, but also our ability to ask it. Need and ability are two quite different matters.

8   *Deserve a response.* Seriousness occurs when decisions need to be made that are humanly significant. A serious question is posed that challenges some aspect of 'practice as usual' (habits, routines). It is serious because we feel obligated to respond. Serious questions are

not simply answered. An interest in the practices of reflection as asking serious questions, brings with it the need for a moral basis of trust and an intellectual basis of struggle within teams. Both demand certain skills, knowledges and sensitivities about the I/me and the us/we. It involves placing our trust in others, trusting that they care and have moral motives. Responding to serious questions demands that we see those with whom we disagree, not as wrong, but as people with important suggestions that need to be carefully considered. Responding to serious questions means we need to be part of a team that is similar enough for meaningful dialogue to happen, but different enough to make it worthwhile. The double-hander of a positive attitude towards diversity within a team (see Part Four) and an ability to search for similarities-within-differences, are processes that fuel an interest in the practices of reflection as asking serious questions.

In a paper on hospital-acquired infections, Davies (2004) gives reasons why nurses should continuously question their practice. The context is that of one in ten patients entering an acute hospital in the UK developing a healthcare-associated infection, of which 9% are wound infections (DoH 2003, 2004). She argues that addressing the problem of hospital-acquired infections requires an improvement in infection control procedures. Questioning practice is the trigger for this. Davies offers the following questions. Which of them do you consider to be 'serious questions'?

- Do we have trolleys dedicated for wound dressings?
- Do we have enough wound-care packs?
- Do we take into a room/cubicle only the equipment/dressings necessary for a particular dressing change?
- Do we have the equipment to enable fluids to be warmed before cleansing wounds?
- Do we change every wound dressing before or just as strike-through occurs?
- Do we always understand the nature of the dressing materials we are using and their purpose, or is it a question of what is available?
- Do we wash our hands?
- Do we educate patients on how to prevent them infecting their own wounds?
- Do we have enough appropriately trained staff to carry out the work?

Plsek *et al.* (2004) asks the following questions. How far would you regard them as serious ones?

- *Relationships.* Do the interactions among the various parts of the system generate energy and innovative ideas for change, or do they drain the organisation?
- *Decision-making.* Are decisions about change made rapidly and by the people with the most knowledge of the issue, or is change bogged down in a treacle of hierarchy and position-authority?

- *Power*. Do individuals and groups acquire and exercise power in positive, constructive ways towards a collective purpose, or is power coveted and used mainly for self-interest and self-preservation?
- *Conflict*. Are conflicts and differences of opinion embraced as opportunities to discover new ways of working, or are these seen as negative and destructive?

What would be some serious questions that arise from reflecting on your own current practice?

Footprints in the spaces-between

The NHS is teeming with teams. For example, we can find project teams, planning teams, quality teams, patient advice and liaison teams, clinical teams. There are uni-professional, integrated and multi-disciplinary teams. Functional and dysfunctional teams. Flat and hierarchical teams. Advisory and action teams. Senior management and ad hoc teams. Real and virtual teams. Leader-led and leader-less teams. Together and fractured teams. Small, middle and large teams. We can find well-developed, embryonic and self-managing teams. Teams whose members all but live and work together, and those that hardly set eyes on each other. Those that work in silos and those that work in the spaces-between. If a team is about 'people doing something together', is it the 'something' that makes the team a team, or is it more to do with the 'being together' part? Maybe it is both and more.

In the section 'Starting Points' I argued that the space-between our customary limits to thinking and practice, can be regarded as a creative space. We need to have the courage to explore this. Teams can be a source of this courage. I remember a primary school teacher of mine saying that I had to draw my lines neatly as wobbly ones simply would not do. I had to learn to draw my letters as carefully as I could. I remember going very slowly on the sides of my 'A', 'A' for Anthony, to make sure they joined up at the top. My teacher did not like wobbly lines. I learnt that I had to colour inside the line and not slide over, outside. She would pick up my colouring if I did, turn it over and walk away saying, 'Start again, too messy'. I sat wondering. Didn't she see my neat lines? Didn't she know I was going to put some sticky dots all over it and make it pretty? And now, much older, how everything seems to be different. Now I have learnt to treat straightness (linearity) with suspicion. The world is indeed fuzzy (wobbly) and we need to learn to work with this not try to control it. Now loose-couplings and virtual networks are important. Now individuals and teams need to be willing to 'colour outside the lines' and not work only from inside a box, a silo, a discipline, and so on.

One final point as we move towards Part Four and address the notion of developing teams. It is about footprints. In a modernising health

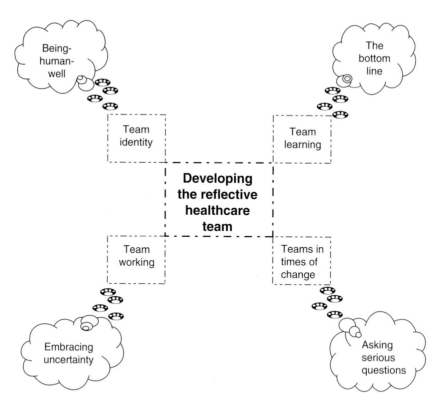

Fig 9.1 Footprints in the spaces-between.

service with all the fuzziness and uncertainty that this brings, it is unwise to be too preoccupied with 'blue-prints'. I suggest we get more preoccupied with 'foot-prints' instead. A blueprint is a kind of answer. In the context of change we have to be prepared to undo 'fast and clean' answers (if indeed these ever existed) and keep asking serious questions. I do not believe there is *a* path, often depicted in 'blue'-prints, only footprints in a sea of sand. What I mean is this. Service improvement and workforce transformation that is responsive to the exigencies of particular situations, may largely have to be invented by teams, along the way. This is different from slavishly following someone else's 'print.' This may sound very scary and irresponsible. But a commitment to the four 'interests' articulated in this part of the book, builds in some safeguards. The practices of reflection help us plot our current position. They enable us to review the steps we have made that have led us to where we are now.

The art of practising reflection helps a team keep track of their thinking and actions. In so doing we give ourselves opportunities for sharing and learning with others who have made similar and different footprints. These prints will always be in sand, as any process of modernisation continually shifts the ground we stand on. The key is to find some relative firmness. Using management of change speak, it is finding the *continuity within the change.* Through the interests and practices of reflection we can make sure our prints are not set in cement and so fixed, immutable and resistant. This is surely a recipe for stress, burnout and exodus as staff. These staff know they have to do things differently, but feel rooted to the spot and unable to do so. These interests in reflection may also provide a compass for us. If we can review the footprints we have made, we may be more able to walk another (and better) way to achieve our goals. We may have to learn to explore what we think we know but also make prints in the emerging spaces-between. Figure 9.1 is therefore an attempt to depict some of the ground in the book so far. How would you 'colour' the space outside the lines? What would you put in the spaces-between? What prints would/can and should your team make?

References

Ackoff, R. (1979) The future of operational research is past. *Journal of Operational Research Society* **30**, 93–104.

Aitkenhead, A. & Slack, J. (1993) *Issues in Cognitive Modelling.* Lawrence Erlbaum, New Jersey.

Argyris, C. & Schön, D. (1992) *Theory in Practice: Increasing Professional Effectiveness.* Jossey Bass, San Francisco.

Ashmore, R. D. & Jussim, L. (eds) (1997) *Self and Identity: Fundamental Issues.* Oxford University Press, New York.

Astor, R., Jefferson, H. & Humphrys, K. (1998) Incorporating the service accomplishments into pre-registration curriculum to enhance reflective practice. *Nurse Education Today* **18**, 567–575.

Atkinson, T. & Claxton, G. (eds) (2000) *The Intuitive Practitioner: On the Value of Not Knowing What One is Doing.* Open University Press, Buckingham.

Bain, J. D., Mills, C., Ballantyne, R. & Packer, J. (2002) Developing reflection on practice through journal writing: impacts of variations in the focus and level of feedback. *Teachers and Teaching: Theory and Practice* **6**(2), 51–73.

Barnett, R. (1997) *Higher Education: A Critical Business.* SRHE & Open University Press, Buckingham.

Bishop, V. (ed) (1998) *Clinical Supervision in Practice: Some Questions, Answers and Guidelines.* Macmillan/NT Research, London.

Bleakley, A. (2000) Writing with invisible ink: narrative, confessionalism and reflective practice. *Reflective Practice* **1**(1), 11–24.

Böhme, G. (2001) *Ethics in Context: The Art of Dealing with Serious Questions.* Polity Press, Cambridge.

Bolton, G. (2001) *Reflective Practice: Writing and Professional Development.* Paul Chapman, London.

Bond, M., & Holland, S. (1998) *Skills of Clinical Supervision for Nurses.* Open University Press, Buckingham.

Brookfield, S. (1990) *The Skillful Teacher.* Jossey Bass, San Francisco.

Bruner, J. (1996) *The Culture of Education.* Harvard University Press.

Burns, S. & Grove, S. (1993) *The Practice of Nursing Research: Conduct, Critique & Utilisation.* Harcourt Brace and Co., Pennsylvania.

Butterworth, T. & Faugier, J. (1997)*Clinical Supervision and Mentorship in Nursing*. Stanley Thornes, Cheltenham.

Butterworth, T., Faugier, J. & Burnard, P. (1998) *Clinical Supervision and Mentorship in Nursing*, 2nd edn. Stanley Thornes, Cheltenham.

Caelli, K. (1998) Shared understandings: negotiating the meanings of health via concept mapping. *Nurse Education Today* **18**, 317–321.

Chesney, M. (1996) Sharing reflections on critical incidents in midwifery practice. *British Journal of Midwifery* **4**(1), 8–11.

Clamp, C. (1980) Learning through Incidents. *Nursing Times*, 2 October, 1755–1758.

Clandinin, D.J. & Connelly, F.M. (1995) *Teachers' Professional Knowledge Landscapes*. Teachers College Press, New York.

Clarke, B., James, C. & Kelly, J. (1996) Reflective practice: reviewing the issues and refocusing the debate. *International Journal of Nursing Studies* **33**(2), 171–180.

Claxton, G. (1999) *Wise Up: the Challenge of Lifelong Learning*. Bloomsbury, London.

Clinton, M. (1998) On reflection in action: unaddressed issues in refocusing the debate on reflective practice. *International Journal of Nursing Practice* **4**(3), 197–202.

Clouder, L. (2000) Reflective practice in physiotherapy education: a critical conversation. *Studies in Higher Education* **25**(2), 211–213.

Coffey, A. & Atkinson, P. (1996) *Making Sense of Qualitative Data*. Sage, London.

Cossentino, J. (2002) Importing artistry: further lessons from the design studio. *Reflective Practice* **3**(1), 39–52.

Covey, S.R. (1999) *The Seven Habits of Highly Effective People: Powerful Lessons in Personal Change*. Simon and Schuster, London.

Crawford, F.R., Dickinson, J. & Leitmann, S. (2002) Mirroring meaning making. *Qualitative Social Work* **1**(2), 170–190.

Daley, B. (1996) Concept maps: linking nursing theory to clinical nursing practice. *The Journal of Continuing Education in Nursing* **27**(1), 17–28.

Davies, P. (2004) Back to the basics of wound care: why nurses should question their practice. *Professional Nurse* **20**(2), 29.

Day, C. (1993) Reflection: a necessary but not sufficient condition for professional development. *British Educational Research Journal* **19**(1), 83–93.

Department of Health (1999) *Making a Difference*. DoH, London.

Department of Health (2003) *Winning Ways: Working Together to Reduce Healthcare Associated Infection in England*. DoH, London.

Department of Health (2004) *Towards Cleaner Hospitals and Lower rates of Infection: a Summary of Action*. DoH, London.

Dewey, J. (1933) *How We Think: a Restatement of the Relation of Reflective Thinking to the Educative Process*. Henrey Regney, Chicago.

Donaghy, M.E. & Morss, K. (2000) Guided reflection: a framework to facilitate and assess reflective practice within the discipline of physiotherapy. *Physiotherapy Theory and Practice* **16**, 3–14.

Durgahee, T. (1997a) Reflective practice: decoding ethical knowledge. *Nursing Ethics* **4**(3), 211–217.

Durgahee, T. (1997b) Reflective practice: nursing ethics through story telling. *Nursing Ethics* **4**(2), 135–146.

Eraut, M. (1995) Schön shock: a case for refraining reflection-in-action? *Teachers and Teaching: Theory and Practice* **1**(1), 9–22.

Errington, E. (ed) (2003) *Developing Scenario-Based Learning: Practical Insights for Tertiary Educators*. Dunmore Press, Palmerston North.

Flannagan, J. (1954) The critical incident technique. *Psychological Bulletin* **51**, 327–358.

Freire P. (1972) *Pedagogy of the Oppressed*. Penguin Books, London.

Freshwater, D. (ed) (2002) *Therapeutic Nursing*. Sage Publications Ltd.

Ghaye, T. (2005) Editorial: reflection for spiritual practice? *Reflective Practice*, **5**(3), 291–295.

Ghaye, T. & Lillyman, S. (1997) *Learning Journals and Critical Incidents*. Quay Books, Mark Allen Publishing Ltd, Dinton.

Ghaye, T. & Lillyman, S. (eds) (1998) *Effective Clinical Supervision: the Role of Reflection*. Quay Books, Mark Allen Group, Dinton.

Ghaye, T. & Lillyman, S. (2000) *Reflection: Principles and Practice for Healthcare Professionals*. Quay Books, Mark Allen Group, Dinton.

Gleick, J. (1991) *Chaos*. Cardinal, Sphere Books.

Glover, P.A. (2000) 'Feedback. I listened, reflected and utilized': third year nursing students' perceptions and use of feedback in the clinical setting. *International Journal of Nursing Practice* **6**(5), 247–252.

Goleman, D. (1997) *Emotional Intelligence: Why it Can Matter More Than IQ*. Bloomsbury, London.

Gould, N. (1996) Introduction: social work education and the 'crisis of the professions'. In *Reflective Learning for Social Work*. (eds N. Gould & I. Taylor). Ashgate, Aldershot.

Graves, S.R. & Addington, T.G. (2002) *Behind the Bottom Line: Powering Business Life with Spiritual Wisdom*. Jossey-Bass, San Francisco.

Haddock, J. (1997) Reflection in groups: contextual and theoretical considerations within nurse education and practice. *Nurse Education Today* **17**(5), 381–385.

Hagland, M. R. (1998) Reflection: a reflex action? *Intensive and Critical Care Nursing: The Official Journal of the British Association of Critical Care Nurses* **14**(2), 96–100.

Hannigan, B. (2001) A discussion of the strengths and weaknesses of 'reflection' in nursing practice and education. *Journal of Clinical Nursing* **10**, 278–283.

Heath, H. (1998) Paradigm dialogues and dogma: finding a place for research, nursing models and reflective practice. *Journal of Advanced Nursing* **28**(2), 288–294.

Heath, H. & Freshwater, D. (2000) Clinical supervision as an emancipatory process: avoiding inappropriate intent. *Journal of Advanced Nursing* **32**(5), 1298–1306.

Higgs, J. & Andresen, L. (2001) The knower, the knowing and the known: threads in the woven tapestry of knowledge. In *Practice Knowledge and Expertise in the Health Professions* (eds J. Higgs & A. Titchen). Butterworth-Heinemann.

Holly, M.L. (1987) *Keeping a Personal-Professional Journal*. Deakin University, Victoria.

Holstein, J. & Gubrium, J. (2000) *The Self we Live by*. Oxford University Press, New York.

Hooks, B. (1995) *Teaching to Transgress: Education as the Practice of Freedom*. Routledge, London.

Hulatt, I. (1995) A Sad Reflection. *Nursing Standard* **9**(20), 22–23.

Irvine, L. (1995) Can concept mapping be used to promote meaningful learning in nurse education? *Journal of Advanced Nursing* **21**, 1175–1179.

Jay, T. (1995) The use of reflection to enhance practice. *Professional Nurse* **10**(9), 593–596.

Johns, C. & Freshwater, D. (eds) (1998) *Transforming Nursing through Reflective Practice*. Blackwell Science, Oxford.

Johns, C. (2000a) *Becoming a Reflective Practitioner*. Blackwell Science, Oxford.

Johns, C. (2000b) Working with Alice: a reflection. *Complementary Therapies in Nursing and Midwifery* **6**, 199–203.

Johns, C. (2001a) Reflective practice: revealing the [He]art of caring. *International Journal of Nursing Practice* **7**(4), 237–245.

Johns, C. (2001b) The caring dance. *Complementary Therapies in Nursing and Midwifery* **7**, 8–12.

Johns, C. (2002) *Guided Reflection: Advancing Practice*. Blackwell Science, Oxford.

Johnson, P. (1969) On the communication of concepts of science. *Journal of Educational Psychology* **58**, 75–83.

Jones, B. & Jones, G. (1996) *Earth Dance Drum: A Celebration of Life*. Commune-A-Key, Salt Lake City.

Kember, D., Jones, A., Loke, A.Y., McKay, J., Sinclair, K., Tse, H., Webb, C., Wong, F.K.Y. & Yeung, E. (2001) *Reflective Teaching and Learning in the Health Professions*. Blackwell Science, Oxford.

Kinsella, E.A. (2001) Reflections on reflective practice. *Canadian Journal of Occupational Therapy* **68**(3), 195–198.

Klemola, U-M. & Norros, L. (2001) Practice-based criteria for assessing anaesthetists' habits of action: outline for a reflexive turn in practice. *Medical Education* **35**(5), 455–464.

Lamont, G. (2002) *The Spirited Business*. Hodder and Stoughton, London.

Loehr, J. & Schwartz, T. (2005) *The Power of Full Engagement: Managing Energy, not Time, is the Key to High Performance and Personal Renewal*. The Free Press.

Loughran, J. & Russell, T. (eds) (2002) *Improving Teacher Education Practices through Self-Study*. RoutledgeFalmer, London.

Love, C. (1996) Critical incidents and prep. *Professional Nurse* **11**(9), 574–577.

MacFarlane, B. (2001) Developing reflective students. *Teaching Business Ethics* **5**(4), 375–387.

Mackintosh, C. (1998) Reflection: a flawed strategy for the nursing profession. *Nurse Education Today* **18**, 553–557.

Maloney, C. & Campbell-Evans, G. (2002) Using interactive journal writing as a strategy for professional growth. *Asia-Pacific Journal of Teacher Education* **30**(1).

Mason, J. (2002) *Researching Your Own Practice: The Discipline of Noticing*. Routledge-Falmer, London.

Mayer, D. (1970) On the representation and retrieval of stored semantic information. *Cognitive Psychology* **1**, 242–299.

McCall, G. & Simmons, J. (1978) *Identities and Interactions*. Free Press, New York.

McCormack, B. (2001) 'The dangers of a missing chapter': a journey of discovery through reflective practice. *Reflective Practice* **2**(2), 209–219.

Miller, D. (1990) *The Icarus Paradox*. Harper Business, New York.

Minghella, E. & Benson, A. (1995) Developing reflective practice in mental health nursing through critical incident analysis. *Journal of Advanced Nursing* **21**, 205–213.

Molloy, J. & Cribb A. (1999) Changing values for nursing and health promotion: exploring the policy context of professional ethics. *Nursing Ethics* **6**(5), 411–421.

Mountford, B. & Rogers, L. (1996) Using individual and group reflection in and on assessment as a tool for effective learning. *Journal of Advanced Nursing* **24**, 1127–1134.

Mullavey-O'Byrne, C. & West, S. (2001) Practising without certainty: providing health care in an uncertain world. In *Professional Practice in Health, Education and the Creative Arts* (eds J. Higgs & A. Titchen). Blackwell Science, Oxford.

Noble, C. (2001) Researching field practice in social work education. *Journal of Social Work* **1**(3), 347–360.

Novak, J. (1998) *Learning, Creating and Using Knowledge*. Lawrence Erlbaum, London.

Nursing Midwifery Council (2002) *Code of Professional Conduct*. NMC, London.

Orland, L. (2000) What's in a line? Exploration of a research and reflection tool. *Teachers and Teaching: Theory and Practice* **6**(2), 197–213.

Paget, T. (2001) Reflective practice and clinical outcomes: practitioners' views on how reflective practice has influenced their clinical practice. *Journal of Clinical Nursing* **10**, 204–214.

Parker, D.L., Webb, J. & D'souza, B. (1995) The value of critical incident analysis as an educational tool and its relationship to experiential learning. *Nurse Education Today* **15**, 111–116.

Parker, S. (1997) *Reflective Teaching in the Postmodern World*. Open University Press, Buckingham.

Peppers, C. & Briskin, A. (2000) *Bringing Your Soul to Work: An Everyday Practice*. Berrett-Koehler.

Peters, T. (1989) *Thriving on Chaos*, 3rd edn. Pan Books, London.

Pinsky, L.E., Monson, D. & Irby, D.M. (1998) How excellent teachers are made. *Advances in Health Sciences Education* **3**(3), 207–215.

Platzer, H., Blake, D. & Ashford, D. (2000) An evaluation of process and outcomes from learning through reflective practice groups on a post-registration nursing course. *Journal of Advanced Nursing* **31**(3), 689–695.

Plsek, P., Bibby, J. & Garrett, S. (2004) *Mapping Behavioural Patterns, Summary Booklet*. NHS Modernisation Agency, London.

Pring, R. (1988) Confidentiality and the right to know. In *Evaluating Education: Issues and Methods* (eds R. Murphy & H. Torrance). Paul Chapman, London.

Pritchard, J. (Ed) (1998) *Good Practice in Supervision*. Jessica Kingsley, London.

Quallington, J. (2000) Ethical reflection: a role for ethics in nursing practice. In *Empowerment through Reflection: The Narratives of Healthcare Professionals* (eds T. Ghaye, D. Gillespie & S. Lillyman). Quay Books, Mark Allen Group, Dinton.

Reid, S. (2002) *How to Think: Building Your Mental Muscle*. Prentice Hall, Pearson Education.

Rich, A. & Parker, D.L. (1995) Reflection and critical incident analysis: ethical and moral implications of their use within nursing and midwifery education. *Journal of Advanced Nursing* **22**, 1050–1057.

Rodgers, C. (2002) Defining reflection: another look at John Dewey and reflective thinking. *The Teachers College Record* **104**(4), 842–866.

Rolfe, G. (2001) Reflective practice: where now? *Nurse Education in Practice* **2**, 21–29.

Rosenfeld, J. & Tardieu, B., (2000) *Artisans of Democracy: How Ordinary People, Families in Extreme Poverty and Social Institutions Become Allies to Overcome Social Exclusion*. University Press of America, Lanham.

Royal College of Nursing (2003) *Clinical Governance: An RCN Resource Guide*. RCN, London.

Samaras, A.P. (2002) *Self-Study for Teacher Educators*. Peter Lang, New York.

Schön, D. (1971) Implementing programs of social and technological change. *Technological Review* **73**(4), 47–51.

Schön, D (1983) *The Reflective Practitioner: How Professionals Think in Action*. New York, Basic Books.

Schön, D (1987) *Educating the Reflective Practitioner: Towards a New Design for Teaching and Learning in the Professions*. Jossey-Bass, San Fransisco.

Schön, D.A. (ed.) (1991) *The Reflective Turn*. Teachers College Press, New York.

Schön, D.A. (1992) The theory of inquiry: Dewey's legacy to education. *Curriculum Inquiry* **22**, 119–39.

Scott, W. (1966) Brief report: measures of cognitive structure. *Multivariate Behavioural Research* **1**(3), 391–395.

Seligman, M. (2004) *Authentic Happiness: Using the New Positive Psychology to Realize your Potential for Lasting Fulfilment*. Nicholas Brealey.

Shavelson, R. (1974) Some methods for examining content structure and cognitive structure in instruction. *Educational Psychologist* **11**(2), 67–85.

Simons, H. & Usher, R. (2000) *Situated Ethics in Educational Research*. Routledge-Falmer, London.

Smith, A. & Russell, J. (1991) Using critical learning incidents in nurse education. *Nurse Education Today* **11**, 284–291.

Smith, B. & Sparkes, A. (2002) Sport, spinal cord injuries, embodied masculinities and the dilemmas of narrative identity. *Men and Masculinities* **4**, 258–285.

Smyth, J. (1991) *Teachers as Collaborative Learners*. Open University Press, Milton Keynes.

Soohbany, M.S. (1999) Counselling as part of the nursing fabric: where is the evidence? A phenomenological study using 'reflection on actions' as a tool for framing the 'lived counselling experiences of nurses'. *Nurse Education Today* **19**, 35–40.

Stake, R. (1995) *The Art of Case Study Research*. Sage, London.

Stewart, I. (1989) *Does God Play Dice?* Blackwell, Oxford.

Stewart, I. (1995) *Nature's Numbers: Discovering Order and Pattern in the Universe*. Weidenfeld and Nicholson, London.

Stewart, I. & Golubitsky, M. (1992) *Complexity: The Emerging Science at the Edge of Order and Chaos*. Simon and Schuster, New York.

Stryker, S. (1994) Freedom and constraint in social and personal life: toward resolving the paradox of self. In *Self, Collective Behaviour and Society: Essays Honouring the Contribution of Ralf H. Turner* (eds G. Platt & C. Gordon), pp. 119–138. JAI Press, Greenwich, Connecticut.

Stuart, C.C. (2001) The reflective journeys of a midwifery tutor and her students. *Reflective Practice* **2**(2), 171–184.

Tajfel, H. (1981) *Human Groups and Social Categories: Studies in Social Psychology*. Cambridge University Press, Cambridge.

Totterdell, M. & Lambert, D. (1999) The professional formation of teachers: a case study in reconceptualising initial teacher education through an evolving model of partnership in training and learning. *Teacher Development* **2**(3), 351–71.

Tripp, D. (1993) *Critical Incidents in Teaching*. Routledge, London.

Turner, J., Hogg, M., Oakes, P. Reicher, S. & Blackwell, M. (1987) *Rediscovering the Social Group; a Self-Categorisation Theory*. Blackwell Publishing, Oxford.

Valkenburg, R. & Dorst, K. (1998) The reflective practice of design teams. *Design Studies* **19**(3), 249–271.

Vince, R. (2002) Organizing reflection. *Management Learning* **33**(1), 63–78.

Wallemaq, A. & Sims, D. (1998) The struggle with sense. In *Discourse and Organisation* (eds D. Grant, T. Keenoy & C. Oswick). Sage, London.

Watson, J. (1999) *Postmodern Nursing and Beyond*. Churchill Livingstone, Edinburgh.

Wheatley, M.J. (1999) *Leadership and the New Science*. Berrett-Koehler, San Francisco.

White, H. (1998) Improving advocacy and partnership: reflection on a critical incident. *Paediatric Nursing* **10**(9), 14–16.

Whitehead, J. (1993) *The Growth of Educational Knowledge: Creating Your Own Living Educational Theories*. Hyde, Bournemouth.

Williams, R.M., Wessel, J., Gemus, M. & Foster-Seargeant, E. (2002) Journal writing to promote reflection by physical therapy students during clinical placements. *Physiotherapy Theory and Practice* **18**(1).

Zollo, J.A. (1998) Reflective practice in nurse education: a step towards equity in education and health care. *Collegian (Royal College of Nursing Australia)* **5**(3), 28–33.

Part Three
About TEAMS: Being the best we can

Chapter 10

What is a team?

Part Two of this book was about *reflection*. It explored some of the interests and practices of it. In this Part, an exploration of the central question, 'How can we develop reflective healthcare teams that are able to sustain high quality, personalised care?' requires an engagement with the literatures about teams.

A lived-experience scenario: how can we work as a team?

Lisa is a team leader for a rapid response team. She recalls:

'As a leader, I wanted to empower my staff to develop a shared vision for the fast response team. The team is multi-professional and includes social workers, occupational therapists, physiotherapists and nurses. I realised that to effectively lead a multi-professional team I would need a much better understanding of the functioning of the staff. While watching the team's dynamics I saw that, despite operating effectively, each profession was functioning separately as 'teams within a team'. The nurses focused predominately on their nurse-led deep vein thrombosis clinic and medical bed management. The social workers and occupational therapist performed patient assessments, which were often collaborative, but the documentation was still distinctly separate.

As a leader, I wanted to empower my staff to develop a shared vision for the fast response team. For effective change to occur, I knew the team would have to move outside their comfort zone. I arranged an 'away day', featuring team building exercises and a chance for discussion about how we should work together. We decided that one of the main objectives would be to enhance our multi-professional working and function as a holistic team. I decided to introduce monthly team meetings with community outside speakers.

One year on, members now say they feel more involved in the decision making process, more motivated and focused. The team also has a shared philosophy and common objectives. The 'teams within a team' syndrome hasn't been completely eradicated, but will continue to be a challenge.'

(Pook 2004, p. 56).

If we reflect on this scenario, there is much to learn. Two particular things are fundamental to this part of the book. I return to them again later. They are *values* and *principles of procedure*. Some of the values embedded in this scenario are that:

1   Individuals benefit from working together and learning how to do so.
2   Working together is complex and difficult at times and requires much commitment and dedication from members.
3   Real teams have mutual perspectives as well as individual ones with separate, sometimes competing and conflicting, interests.
4   Teams (and teams-within-teams) frequently have overlapping interests, areas of expertise, strengths and limitations.
5   It is important to appreciate similarities-within-difference. That in a team, there are staff who are no different from one another. There are others who also (like you) have feelings, a sense of humour, sensitivities, an individual spirit, aspirations and a way of seeing the world.
6   If we can change the context (for team learning) we stand a chance of changing behaviour and therefore the way teams work (Gladwell 2000).
7   Staff rarely change their practice through the rational process of *analyse-think-change*. They are much more likely to change in a *see-feel-change* process (Kotter & Cohen 2002).

Some principles of procedure we sense in this scenario are;

a   The need to invest time in understanding each profession's/discipline's value positions, in negotiating shared concerns and reaching a shared vision for a team's future work.
b   The need to create opportunities for teams to acknowledge and internalise their own capacity to learn about ways to erode 'separateness'. Only then is it likely that staff see their responsibility to overcome it.
c   Being clear about the role of the team leader to provide an enabling context for staff to 'see' new possibilities. For team leaders, it may be hard to refuse those who place their hope in you!
d   Appreciating a team's progress over time and celebrating a team's achievements.
e   Using particular team development activities that: (a) *Encourage* members to become actively involved in decisions about services. This means staff do not attend team meetings as 'mere spectators' but are actively encouraged to take part and learn whatever they can from others. (b) *Embrace* diversity of staff views positively and help develop a shared language and one that is not patronising to anyone. (c) *Empower* team members to continuously aspire to utilise the benefits of multi-professional working for the benefit of patients, clients and families. With greater feelings of empowerment come more possibilities to act. Armed with this, staff can begin to sense that there actually are choices. That there is a margin of freedom to take a stand on service issues or not.
f   Working to create protected learning time that helps sustain good team working. This also serves to cultivate a sense of community which creates, shares and applies knowledge and expertise to practice (Wenger *et al.* 2002).

In general the major books on the subject of teams, over the last decade, have remained basically upbeat and have focused primarily on how to develop teams successfully. But there have been books with a more cautious and qualified approach. Three examples are: *Why Teams Fail and What to do About it* (Hitchcock & Willard 1995), *Why Teams Don't Work: What Went Wrong and How to Make it Right* (Robbins & Finley 1995) and *Team Traps: Survival Stories and Lessons from Team Disasters, Near-Misses, Mishaps, and Other Near-Death Experiences* (Rayner 1996). Each of these books focused on practical problems that were associated with team development. In spite of their emphasis on problems these texts remained upbeat about the overall applicability of team efforts with the caveat that team development be 'done right'.

Dream teams

Dr and Mrs Lundin are business partners at Psychological Dynamics in Wisconsin, USA. They work with organisations on team building and culture change. Part of an account of one of their workshops is described here (Lundin & Lundin 1996, p. 119):

'The Vice President attended a two-day retreat on team building. During the flight back he tingled from the good fellowship and stimulating ideas. He hummed themes from the rousing musical finale, the 1812 Overture. Back at work he announced. 'We need teams. We're being left behind.' You are appointed a team leader. Great things are expected of team leaders. The retreat promised dream teams.

A week after the Vice President's return, corporate matters were in his face, the tingling had disappeared and Tchaikovsky was forgotten. But he still had the task to develop a dream team, make the members tingle and inspire them to produce.'

This may be a familiar experience for many. Some describe it as a reality shock. We get 'back to base' and all the enthusiasm and great ideas we have seem to take on a different hue. What's possible seems suddenly to be less so. What is essential suddenly falls into a 'merely desirable' box. What can be done transforms into a maybe. What needs to be tackled today is put off until later. So I wonder how we get from a memory to a lived reality? The Lundin's have their own theory. It goes like this (Lundin & Lundin 1996, p. 119):

'The Vice President has to stop long enough to observe his own behaviour and save his staff a lot of heartache. You can't copy another team's inspiration. It wasn't them who tingled or heard the inspired music. In addition;

- *Inspiration wears off*
- *It's the doing, not the speeches, that matters*
- *Musicians get tired*
- *There's a long time between peak experiences*

The pathway to a dream team will lead you through those grinding, grating, often frightening, sometimes smooth and harmonious, uplifting interfaces of life – the emotions. Some will say through our souls, others through our hearts. We prefer to say through our relationships . . . the real thing with their irregular outlines and messy edges'.

Dream teams are only one kind of team. For some a fantasy, others a reality. Fundamentally, when we talk about a healthcare team, we must not assume that the word means the same thing to everyone. Just think for a moment about the different ways you, yourself, describe teams. Maybe ones you have been a part of, worked with and encounter each day. There is, of course, a difference between how we might describe ourselves and how others might see us. I have heard teams describe themselves as a district nursing team, a paediatric occupational therapy team, a team of radiographers, an administrative and support team, a team of medical consultants in oncology, a team of social workers, dentists, and so on. This is one way of describing a team. It is to portray ourselves as people who have some things in common. In this instance and in general terms, it is something about what they all do. A multidisciplinary team have things in common also. But this may be regarded as a different kind of team to those just listed. Why?

I have also heard teams describe themselves as community mental health teams, a team of prison nurses, a team working in an acute hospital, a hospice, a hospital at home team. This adds an additional descriptive layer. It tells us something about where people most often work. But what about those who work for twilight and evening services, or those who describe themselves as working 'school term time' only? Maybe this says something about when people work? And what about a team of senior managers, a locality manager's team, a clinical leader team? What does this say to us? Are these teams defined by role, responsibility, experience, aptitude, seniority, merit? Maybe one or more attributes. Others? You may feel descriptors like 'moving', 'cruising', 'struggling' or even 'sinking' might be closer to your own experience of team working!

Being the best we can

Collins' (2001) analyses of 1435 companies that appeared in *Fortune 500* from 1965–1995 and that went from good to great, is a catalyst for thinking about the process of developing 'great' teams in the NHS. Although Collins relied on a single measure of success, namely financial performance, his three core themes for success are very useful. They are those of:

1 disciplined people;
2 disciplined thought; and
3 disciplined action.

Table 10.1 Being the best we can (summary of Collins 2001).

Build up	Breakthrough	Being the best we can
Disciplined people is about **level 5 leadership**	**Disciplined thinking** is about **confronting the brutal facts**	**Disciplined action** is about **sustaining a culture of discipline**
(e.g. A blend of personal humility with professional will) and **getting the right people** then developing **new vision and strategy**	(e.g. What needs improving) and **deciding on organisational priorities**	(e.g. Autonomy with Responsibility) and **using modern technologies**
(e.g. People-first then direction)	(e.g. How do we meet our targets?)	(e.g. National Programme for IT in the NHS)

Table 10.1 sets these themes out in more detail.

1 *Disciplined people*. Collins (2001) found that the type of leaders needed for moving staff from being good, to being great, were generally self-effacing, quiet, reserved, even shy. A paradoxical blend of personal humility and professional will. More like Lincoln and Socrates than Patton and Caesar. So not high profile leaders with big personalities who make the headlines. I return to this later when I discuss 'quiet leadership'. He also found the good-to-great process began with getting the 'right' staff in the 'right' places within the organisation, then using this talent to set about developing visions and strategies.

2 *Disciplined thought*. One aspect of this is that staff must be clear about their commitments to providing the very highest quality service and maintain this through times of difficulty and challenge. At the same time Collins found that staff need to confront the realities of the situations they find themselves in. To confront the brutal facts of these situations, whatever they may be. This not only takes clarity of thinking but also courage, passion and a process of service improvement that works (see Part Four). The other part of disciplined thought is about clarifying the way staff think about: (a) What is it we are passionate about? (b) What can we be best at? (c) What is most viable?

3 *Disciplined action*. Interestingly, Collins (2001) argues that all organisations have workplace cultures and some work in very disciplined

ways. But few have a *culture* of discipline. Discipline is given a very positive spin. He says that when organisations have disciplined staff, they do not need hierarchy. When staff use disciplined thinking, they do not need to rely on bureaucracy. When organisations have disciplined action, they do not need excessive controls. In Part Four of this book I describe a form of disciplined action that has been developed with staff and service users in healthcare. It has five mutually supporting elements and is called TA^{2}LK (IRP-UK 2005). The elements of disciplined action it embraces are:

T ... echnology-enabled learning

It uses modern technology to support staff and service users to identify key areas for action to improve practice and policy.

A ... ccelerated results

It helps build positive team improvement plans, for quick wins, by enabling staff and service users to think and act differently.

A ... ccessible process

TA^{2}LK is an inclusive process of transformational improvement. It therefore has to be accessed by and impact on, a critical mass of staff. In this way everyone in the organisation can be aligned to its vision and be held accountable in meaningful ways.

L ... asting impact

It works to ensure that a team's transformational improvement efforts are not 'flavour of the month' but are lasting and sustainable.

K ... nowledge sharing

Through facilitated reflective conversations, this disciplined action enables teams to manage their talent, learn and work much better together.

With regard to technology (the T of TA^{2}LK), Collins found that staff who engage with this good-to-great process think about the role of technology differently (see Langer's 2005 influential work also). They are pioneers in the application of carefully selected technologies. The National Programme for IT in the NHS in the UK, could be regarded as an example of this. The aim of the National Programme is to bring modern computer systems into the NHS to improve patient care and services. Over the next 10 years it will connect over 30 000 GPs in England to almost 300 hospitals and give patients access to their personal health and care information, transforming the way the NHS works. Information will move around more quickly with healthcare records, appointments, prescription information and up-to-date research into illnesses and treatments, accessible to patients and health professionals whenever they need it.

Talk about teams

Developing teams is a complicated process. A fundamental question is: What kind of team do you want to develop? The follow-up question then becomes: How can you do this, in a disciplined and supportive manner, in the circumstances? Disciplined thought is required to answer the first question. Disciplined people and action, the second. The development process does not often present us with a clean sheet of paper to work on. Occasionally we can indeed develop new teams from scratch. But most of the time we work with existing staff teams (and groups), trying to enable them to do something else or develop into something different! A relatively recent and challenging example of both of these things is the development of intermediate care teams. Sometimes effort and resources is given over to develop 'troubled teams' into more harmonious and effective ones. The development of 'effective' teams, 'high performing', 'great' or 'modern' teams for a modern NHS, requires different kinds of disciplined thinking, people and actions.

A team might share a common client base or case load, a common 'patch' where they work. They may share more subtle things like a common experience of working under pressure, with poor facilities or in relative isolation. Members might share a common sense of history 'Where we've come from and what we've been through', a common set of values that provide good reasons for 'Doing what we do, this way'; maybe a shared sense of hope, optimism and commitment to lifelong learning. Sometimes staff may be part of one or more teams, a dysfunctional team, 'dream' team or no team at all! These things and more add to the complexity of the development process.

A clinical governance support team

Both the complexity and expansiveness of team development in the NHS can be illustrated with reference to an advertisement, jointly posted by the UK's NHS Modernisation Agency and Department of Health in 2003 for a 'team coach'. A central purpose of this role was described thus:

'To develop effective team working which produces continuous improvements in the delivery of patient care by:

- creating an open but challenging blame-free culture;
- supporting multi-disciplinary and multi-agency teamworking;
- supporting teams around identified care pathways.'

The preamble to the job description read:

'This is a unique opportunity to make a noticeable and personal impact on creating a better NHS. Acting as an internal consultant, you will drive cultural and organisational change and create an open, but challenging blame-free culture in which multi-discipline, multi-agency teams can deliver continuous improvements in patient care... where teams are troubled or dysfunctional, you will go in, find out what is going on, identify the causes and underlying issues, provide advice, guidance and interventions – often one-to-one work within the organisation... and then move on to the next challenge as soon as the time is right.'

One cluster of team coach competencies came under a heading called 'promoting teamwork'. The cluster stated that the coach:

'Helps develop empowered, flexible and cohesive teams within and across organisations, directorates, departments and functions,
- identifies personally with organisational and team objectives;
- promotes collaborative and co-operative ways of working;
- encourages others to make their contribution to effective team working;
- develops teams to manage potential conflicts between individual team members;
- works as an effective team member in a variety of teamwork contexts;
- works as an effective team member with a wide variety of different individuals in differently composed teams.'

The challenge of this post, conveyed in the language (content, tone and tenor) used, is certainly not one for the faint hearted. One reading of this advert is a view that teams can work better with the help of a coach that can assess and diagnose the context in which a team is working, get things sorted, work in and on the team and the organisation and then get out and move on to the next challenge! The cultural context in which a team works is stressed. This is to be applauded. Rather more worrying is the use of a motoring metaphor, in the advert, to describe a process of building a culture where, '... multi-discipline, multi-agency teams can deliver continuous improvements in patient care'. 'Driving' cultural and organisational change is a dangerous, even inappropriate, business and is in an uneasy juxtaposition, in the same competence cluster, with expressions of developing more empowered teams. I have no problems with the use of metaphor, in general. The key issue is which metaphor we choose and how far it helps us understand a complex process. Interestingly, and in contrast, a team leader for a large, 35-member intermediate care team revealed in conversation:

'I don't think I can push, persuade, cajole or bully the team into anything. We've got to go at the pace we feel is right for us. We can't rush things. We are quite newly formed, you see, so we need time to talk to each other and sort out what's important to us, what our service is about, what we can do. And my role ... well ... it's an interesting and challenging one. Some want me to lead from the front... to tell them... about this and that. I can do this if this is what they really need. But I have staff who are very good and have their own views. They are very experienced in what they do. I have to acknowledge this... use it... you know foster it. And I feel uncomfortable taking the lead all the time. I don't think it's right either. Maybe all they need is a gentle nudge from time to time. You see you've got to read the signs. Feel the vibes. Sense what's in the air. Don't push and drive things on at breakneck speed . . . we are under pressure of course . . . but I just feel this will be our undoing later I think. Just a light touch on the tiller . . . you know, a bit like sailing a boat well.'

(With thanks to Joan, in conversation with Tony, 20 February 2003)

Arguably even more worrying is that the advert makes no reference at all to any expression of the power and potency of 'reflection' or to *team learning*. This is a fundamental omission. There are of course multiple readings of this advert. How do you read it? How far do you feel that the underlying story here is of an energetic, visionary government with zero tolerance of failure to respond to its vision of team working? Perhaps this is too harsh. But the silences regarding the practices of reflection, and *teams-that-learn* is problematic. For example, how would any kind of team know how far it was achieving 'continuous improvements in the delivery of patient care' if there was no culture of reflection within it? I take the practice of reflection here to mean the systematic, rigorous and public (team-generated and team-discussed) reflection on its delivery of patient care. I am sure the practices of reflection are a part of the support team's work. In an interim report (Dawson & Smith 2002, p. v) evaluating the impact of clinical governance support teams, reflection is given as an important indication of a 'group's ability to learn'.

From loose staff groups to teams that perform

There are many kinds of healthcare teams, doing different, and in some cases, complementary things. Teams also work in a particular context which have particular workplace cultures. These influence what a team feels, thinks and can do. What staff do, how they do it and in what context is illustrated by Scott (2003, p. 662).

'In the pages of *Professional Nurse* we talk about many nurse-led initiatives that drive forward the quality of patient care – new roles, new services, the application of evidence-based research and different methods of organisation, for example. But this is only part of the picture. Without enough staff or the right balance of skills and experience no nursing team can operate efficiently, let alone begin to think about working in different ways. The reality is of increased workload, job vacancies and high use of temporary staff . . . The Audit Commission (2002) found that, of the people who leave the NHS, nearly half do so for less pay – an incredible statistic. So although Agenda for Change is expected to give a positive boost to many salaries in the future, pay is not thought to be the main issue. What is key is that people feel happy in their jobs, challenged and appreciated. Trusts who have invested time and effort in offering good training and development are leading the way in terms of providing a supportive and stimulating place to work'

In discussions about teams, fundamental questions to ask are:

(a)   What is a team?
(b)   How does a team work?
(c)   How do its members learn?
(d)   How far is it working well?

In the context of evidence-based practice, another question is:

(e)   What evidence have I got about the performance of this team in achieving its goals?

Additional questions are:

(f)   Why does this group of people call itself a team?
(g)   How do teams cope with fluctuating membership?
(h)   Should we define a team by the people who are part of it, by what it does or by what it stands for?
(i)   What are service users' views of the question: What is a good team?
(j)   How far is being a part of a team a source of human-well-being and/or a resource for struggle?

Accepting that a team-based philosophy is an appropriate mechanism for facilitating effective service delivery, is also to accept that teams enable staff to be competent and confident when they work together. Clearly this is not true on the first day that a new team is assembled. Loose groups of individuals do not transform into an effective team instantaneously, or randomly. There are processes at work that take time to play out. Sheard and Kakabadse (2002) studied the processes by which a loose group of staff transformed into an effective team. They drew upon the work of Tuckman (1965), who described four stages in the development of a team. They are forming, storming, norming and performing stages. Additionally, they drew on the work of Kübler Ross (1969), who studied the dynamics of personal transition and change.

Sheard and Kakabadse (2002) formulated an *integrated team-development framework*, which highlights nine key factors that collectively differentiate a loose group from an effective team (see Table 10.2). The framework comprises four basic elements, namely: task, individual, group and environment. The basic element called *task* relates specifically to the goal which a team is required to deliver. Without a task to perform, a group of individuals has no reason to transform into a team at all, and therefore will remain no more than a collection of individuals. The second key factor associated with *task* is priorities. They called the second basic element the *individual* and broke it down into two parts. One called roles and responsibilities, the other self-awareness. What is relevant here is the individual's ability to foresee the consequences of their actions and behaviour. This is particularly important for good team learning and working. The third basic element called *group* embodies those aspects of team working that are derivative of the team's ability to function as a unit.

Table 10.2 The nine key factors for an integrated team development framework. Source: Summary of Sheard and Kakabadse (2002).

Basic element	Key factor	Loose group	Effective team
Task	Clearly defined goals	Individuals opt out if goals not understood	Understood by all
Task	Priorities	Split loyalty of individuals to other groups	Cohesive team alignment
Individual	Roles and responsibilities	Unclear, with gaps and overlap	Agreed and understood by individuals
Individual	Self-awareness	Individuals guarded	Behaviour appropriate to team needs
Group	Leadership	Directive	Catalytic
Group	Group dynamics	Individuals guarded	Social system established and accepted
Group	Communications	Formal	Open dialogue
Environment	Content	Task focused	Influenced, but not controlled, by organisation
Environment	Infrastructure	Task focused	Stable support from organisational infrastructure

The first key factor identified is leadership. The second is group dynamics. This is saying that a team needs to be seen as being more than simply a collection of individuals working towards a common goal. It is also a social system. The third key factor is communication. The last basic element called *environment* has two parts: infrastructure and context.

During the construction of their integrated team-development framework, Sheard & Kakabadse (2002) were able to clarify what was significant in the transformation of a loose group into an effective team. This led them to formulate a team development process, which they named the *team landscape*, as it comprised the landscape through which a team must navigate during its transformation.

Some relevant findings are thus:

- When teams are first formed the single most significant aspect that contributes to their development is the clarity of their goal/s.

Members need to know why they are called a team, what their purposes are and what binds them together. This is related to a clarification of the team's values and thereby what it stands for. A goal-planning process, involving all team members, results in a very much more coordinated team.

- At the next stage, understanding team dynamics becomes critical. This was what James (1999) referred to as the process of creating a social system where previously there was none. Excellent communication associated with close member support, was concluded to assist in the development of a supportive team social structure. Rushmer (1997) expresses this as the processes of staff 'speaking to' and 'getting to know' each other. We can also understand this in terms of Maslow's theory of motivation (Maslow 1987), in that team members derive satisfaction for their safety and belongingness needs from membership of the team. On closer examination of Rushmer's (1997) work we find that there is more to this *getting to know each other*, than simply socialising. It involves a task-oriented element. He found that staff also got to know the strengths and weaknesses of other team members and how to work with these within the team.

- With these addressed and understood, team development then begins to centre upon leadership issues. Leadership (as a set of processes) was found to be the single most important part of the team development landscape. With regard to leaders (not leadership) the ability of a team leader to communicate effectively and find workable common ground that all team members accept, were seen to be key skills. There was also clear evidence to indicate that the formally appointed team leader performed better with the close support of others in what can be characterised as supporting roles.

- The links between the whole organisation (environment) and the performance of a team are subtle ones. An important one is for 'management' to avoid doing anything that stops the team from performing. Sheard & Kakabadse (2002) found that once teams were performing, they were routinely stopped from doing so by senior management in four ways: (1) changing priorities at short notice; (2) removing key team members for 'important' jobs elsewhere; (3) allowing teams to fall apart by simply removing members until there are none left and never formally disbanding them; and (4) informing the team leaders what to do and in so doing disempowering them.

- The links between team work and the whole organisation can also be described as one of *alignment*. For teams to perform well two basic things have to be aligned. They are values and staff commitment to them. Gladwell (2002) asserts that one of the lessons of the debacle of Enron is that even if the best and the brightest people are formed into teams and given virtually unlimited authority, they may not automatically produce positive results for the organisation. Enron hired the highest-achieving students from top business schools, and provided them with plentiful financing, other tools and resources. But in the end the firm declared bankruptcy and executives were charged with fraud. Teams accelerated the decline of the firm because they did not have a commitment to the organisation. They were focused on personal gain and not on long-term results. They did not have agreed goals, roles, responsibilities and priorities. Eggensperger (2004) calls this 'missing work ethics'.

- A peer review process of team's performance, after they had worked towards achieving a particular goal, facilitated transformation. Review would be an opportunity for staff to present what they had achieved, the processes used and the evidence to support their claims.
- Interestingly, they emphasise the impact of leadership on both the ability of a staff group to transform into a team and the speed with which it does so. Specifically, the greater the team members' personal confidence in the quality of team leadership the shorter the transformation time from group to team.

When team members try to enhance their performance Kipp & Kipp (2000) suggest that staff are not well served by any process that 'psychotherapises' individual members – publicly or one by one. Serial executive coaching, they argue, is not teambuilding. They also state that removing 'bad apples', while sometimes long overdue, may not alter a team's group dynamics. It may just create a vacancy if the underlying patterns of relationships are left unaddressed. Time together is often linked with team development. They say that of itself, time changes nothing. Teams that have been together for years are often no more effective than when they started, unless they have worked on how they learn and work together. Their last point genuinely opens up some new ground. They say that performing as a team is about *emotional maturity* and that there is no substitute for this (Kipp & Kipp 2000, p. 139). In Part Four of this book I place this in the broader frame of a team's *emotional literacy* and argue how it is an essential attribute of a reflective healthcare team.

When checking on the ability of a team to 'perform' the Kipp and Kipp (2000, p. 138) six-point list is a useful summary. They suggest staff reflect upon their:

1 *Goals.* What constitutes 'success' for us, in this situation and overall?
2 *Roles.* What is expected of us? What do we expect of each other?
3 *Rules.* What are our agreements on decision making and work ethic?
4 *Relationships.* How do we handle conflict, ambiguity, rumour, secrecy and trust?
5 *Results.* How do we determine how well we are performing day to day?
6 *Rewards.* What is in it for us – individually and collectively? Are we 'OK' with that?

Reflecting on some customary thinking about teams

If we need to change the things that matter, we need to listen to those who know what matters most. This means accessing and understanding relevant and meaningful knowledge about teams and managing this well. Staff cannot be told they are now a team and then be expected to act like one (Rabey 2001). Working well in a team takes time. In concluding this section I offer you six broad themes that might enable teams to be the best they can. They are:

- *Team learning and team work.* What do you want the word team to mean in your workplace and in the context of a modernising National Health Service?
- *The centrality of values.* What do you want your team to stand for?
- *The individual vis-à-vis the team.* How can you learn to share and share to learn?
- *Knowledge.* Whose knowledge counts and how is this knowledge most appropriately managed and shared within and between teams (McIntyre 2003)?
- *Conversation.* How do you sustain team conversations that are not ones of blame, but of constructive critique, hopefulness and possibility?
- *Serious questions.* What is a modern team for a modern health service?

Chapter 11

Team learning and team work = Team*ability*

An important outcome of good team learning and working is what a team is able to achieve. This is summarised in the form of a team*ability* 'triangle' and shown in Fig. 11.1.

A team's functioning capability is its *ability* to achieve a certain goal and/or perform particular tasks. To do this team members need both knowledge and skill. An equally important component of team *ability* is *will* and principally what values team members are choosing to commit to and deliver against. This is also about what kinds of difference (to services) the team wishes to make. This will inevitably involve the careful management of resistance. Team's also have a *state of being*. This encapsulates what the team's culture is like. More about this later.

What is a high performing team?

A team's performance is certainly a dominant strand of work in the field. This includes identifying the variables critical for team effectiveness (Flory 1998, Fleming & Monda-Amaya 2001), the management and prediction of performance (Jackson 2002, Telleria *et al.* 2002) and the relationships between team performance and organisational cultures (Boaden & Leaviss 2000, Castka *et al.* 2003). Rickards & Moger (1999) call high performing teams 'dream teams' and define seven attributes that distinguish them from 'teams from hell'. They are:

1   a strong platform of understanding;
2   a shared vision;
3   a creative climate;
4   an ownership of ideas;
5   a resilience to setbacks;
6   a network of activators; and
7   they learn from reflecting on experience.

Authors (Peters & Waterman 1982, Imai 1986, Nonaka & Takeuchi 1995, Stott & Walker 1995) all argue that an environment of tolerance towards failures and mistakes and a certain amount of creative chaos can do much to improve team performance.

Team performance is also the thrust of the work of Katzenbach & Smith (2003) as described in their book *The Wisdom of Teams*. They advance a view that teams and performance are inextricably connected. In their

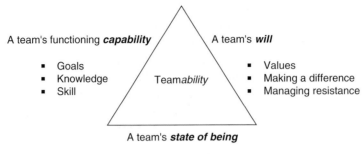

A team's functioning **capability**

- Goals
- Knowledge
- Skill

Team*ability*

A team's **will**

- Values
- Making a difference
- Managing resistance

A team's **state of being**

- Physical resilience (work-rest ratio)
- Emotional literacy
- Realistic optimism
- Fitness-for-purpose

Fig 11.1   A Team*ability* triangle.

work they try to explain why they believe there is confusion about what a team is and also confusion over what helps to make teams perform well. They talk about the need to get the 'basics' right if we are to nurture a particular kind of team. The one they have in mind is the 'high-performance' team. These are, '... *real teams ... deeply committed to their purpose, goals and approach. High performance team members are also very committed to one another ... However meaningful, 'team' is always a result of pursuing a demanding performance challenge*' (Katzenbach & Smith 2003, p. 9). In summary their 'team basics' are a collective concern with the skills members have or need, their commitment to commonly known and shared purposes and collective accountability. This allows them to go on and offer a generic definition of a team. They stress that this definition distinguishes a team from a group of people. They also stress that groups become teams through 'disciplined action'. '*A team is a small number of people with complementary skills who are committed to a common purpose, performance goals, and approach for which they hold each themselves mutually accountable*' (Katzenbach & Smith 2003, p. 45).

Interestingly they argue that '... *performance outcomes and results must be the primary objective in choosing the team approach, not the desire to be a team*' (Katzenbach & Smith 2003, p. xviii). They claim that the single most powerful engine for teams is a clear and compelling performance challenge. They believe teams are much more about performance than togetherness. I will question this in Part Four of this book. I have come to believe that a sense of togetherness and performance are linked in some important ways. Interestingly, what they call 'team discipline' is central to their view of creating a high performance organisation. They go on to state that 'other aspects of teaming' (such as openness and communication) remain important but that these are not as critical as their 'six basics'. In this book I take issue with the way these 'other aspects' appear to make an important, but not an essential contribution, to being a team. Later I will explain how recent evidence suggests that some 'other aspects' are indeed essential.

Team building is not just a cognitive process and 'team coaches' of the kind described earlier, are not car mechanics, fixing things when they go wrong. Nurturing good team learning and working rests upon the sensitive handling and deployment of positive emotions, of feelings and relationships (Amason *et al.* 1995, Polley & Ribbens 1998). Sometimes we need to relearn the obvious, and for some, the obvious qualities that constitute a team are a faith in oneself, trust in team members and an optimism about the future. We will have a look at these in more detail in Part Four.

What makes a team effective?

In the work of Fleming and Monda-Amaya (2001) we find an interesting list of process variables critical for team effectiveness. These include team goals, team membership and roles, team communication, team cohesion, team logistics and team outcomes. Team goals, outcomes and cohesion were seen to be the most critical to team effectiveness. It is in their category of team cohesion that we find some very important variables that I will return to later. Specifically, they are to do with trust, support and decision-making. The category comprised:

- Members feel safe sharing ideas
- The team has trust among members
- Members feel equally empowered
- The team has a unified goal
- The team has time to celebrate
- The team has support from superiors
- Members have respect for each other
- The team has recognition for efforts
- The team has autonomy for decision making
- The team has a healthy regard for disagreement

(Fleming & Monda-Amaya, 2001, p. 168).

Reflecting on the multi-professional team

This kind of teamwork, as a preferred approach to practice, has been promoted for many areas of healthcare by policy makers, professional bodies and Trust management (Calman & Hine 1995, DoH 1997, 1998, SCOPME 1997, Freeman & Procter-Childs 1998). The study by Freeman and Procter-Childs (1998) was supported by the English National Board and had two aims. First, to try to identify the skills and knowledge required by students to work effectively in a multi-professional team. Second, to examine current educational provision to prepare students for this kind of team working. Using a case study design, they explored issues around professional interaction that appeared to inhibit or support this way of team working. Six teams comprised the study. They were a diabetes team, a primary healthcare team, a medical ward team, a neuro-rehabilitation team, child development assessment team and community mental health team. During the conduct of the study they became aware that individual professionals had very different views of 'effective multi-professional teamwork' and that this inhibited professionals from working effectively together. They state, 'Individual philosophies of team-working seemed to shape perceptions of the need for shared vision, what constituted effective communication and role understanding, and how role contribution was valued. In relation to these, the different philosophies led to different expectations of learning from other team members' (Freeman & Procter-Childs 1998, p. 241). The philosophies were labelled as 'directive', 'integrative' and 'elective'. Their essential attributes were found to be thus.

- *The directive philosophy*. This was a prevalent view most frequently held by medical staff. It is a philosophy where team learning is influenced by status and the real and perceived power relations between colleagues. Team working is conditioned by different kinds of hierarchy. A team leader is appointed on the basis of status and power. The nature of communication between staff is determined by what the 'leader' thinks is significant. Those who feel of 'lower status' tend to find it hard to question the status quo. Very significantly, '... the philosophy made assumptions about understanding others' roles in terms of tasks. Where roles were lower in the hierarchy, they were valued for their service to the powerful role rather than having an intrinsic value in terms of insights into patient care' (Freeman & Proctor-Childs 1998, p. 241). From this description it is hard to deter-mine what, other than the exercising of power and the suffocation of individual expression and creativity, actually held teams like this together.

- *The integrative philosophy*. Freeman & Procter-Childs (1998) found that this was prevalent amongst therapists, approved social workers and held by some nursing staff. At the heart of this philosophy is a commitment to the practice of collaborative care and therapy, to being a team player, an understanding that members of the team may have different roles and the importance of negotiated role boundaries. Importantly, each member's unique contribution to the team is valued. There is an optimistic acknowledgement that mem-bers would indeed learn skills and knowledge from each other.

- *The elective philosophy*. They found that this was held most often by staff working in mental health services. The key defining attribute of this philosophy was an insularity of practice. *'Professionals who pre-ferred to operate autonomously and referred to other professionals as and when they perceived there was a need'* (Freeman & Proctor-Childs

1998, p. 214). This takes us back, once again, to earlier notions of cultures of individualism and separation. Freeman & Procter-Childs (1998) allude to this when they refer to role distinctiveness, '... *brevity of communication in order only to inform others*' and lack of sharing through the withholding of case notes. Again it is somewhat difficult to confidently describe staff, who subscribe to this philosophy, as team players contributing to better team learning and working.

So what are some of the general implications of this work? First, this is a further example of the multiplicity of meanings conveyed by the word 'team' and the difficulties and opportunities that arise from differently held views. We may have an intellectual debate about the different meanings associated with 'multi-professional' and multi-disciplinary' teams (Lowe & O'Hara 2000, Boaden & Leaviss 2000), between inter-professional team working (Elston & Holloway 2001) and sustaining inter-professional collaboration' (Freeth 2001). It should not be a question of semantics. The serious and defining talk is about what these teams actually do and what they stand for. Second, it is important to be clear about which conception of 'team' staff have in their minds. It is not wise to assume that everyone is holding the same view. In NHS organisations we sometimes naively think that we speak the same language, when in reality organisations, to a greater or lesser extent, are little towers of Babel. Third, how we think about the word 'team' influences how we behave in a team. For example, Freeman & Procter-Childs (1998) found that this shaped how and what staff communicated with each other.

A lived scenario: multi-disciplinary team working

'The closure both of a long-term institution for young disabled adults and an elderly care hospital necessitated a review ... of how therapy services could best be provided for the former residents when they moved into the community. There appeared to be two options. The first was to extend the current uni-disciplinary model of provision into the community. This would mean that provision would be based on services organised according to professional groupings. Each would allocate a proportion of their total hours' budget to provide for the former residents when they moved. The second option was to create multi-disciplinary teams (MDTs) of clinicians, who would be responsible for delivering the full range of services to particular client groups. With this way of working staff would be managed, not according to professional groups, but according to the client groups that they served' *(Lowe & O'Hara, 2000, p. 269).*

One major outcome from the problem scenario was that the introduction of multi-disciplinary team working meant that all those involved had to fundamentally reappraise their role and '... relinquish their attachment to their own disciplines' (Lowe & O'Hasa 2000, p. 278). This is a very significant finding in relation to the broader issue of both personal and professional identity. Arguably, for many staff, it is an attachment to their discipline that gives them a real sense of professional identity, self-worth and esteem. This is a big concern for some. It is a way one 'positions' oneself in relation to another. The way we present our professional identities to others (e.g. I am a doctor, I am a psychologist, and so on) gives rise to particular kinds of conversation. It may stifle others, particularly if the identity being articulated is regarded as 'different'.

It is fair to say that the development of personal and collective (team) identities is a complex and important process. For some staff, being part of a team brings with it an erosion of personal identity. If we see or regard ourselves in a particular way, like a speech and language therapist, or a community midwife, then we act, or try to act, in a way congruent with this. Then there are the publicly presented personas of team members as they engage with other professionals and service users. Individual and team identities are linked to an important body of ideas called positioning theory (Harré & Langenhove 1999). Being part of a team does not necessarily mean that personal and professional identities have to be relinquished or compromised. This is a fear some staff have. They may in fact be enhanced and nourished. Much depends upon what matters most, to whom and why?

Another major conclusion of the work of Lowe and O'Hara (2000, p. 278) is expressed thus, *'Managers have had to abandon their traditional model of managing. All have had to develop new skills and attitudes that fit the new way of working'*. This opens up a vital area for further reflection. I will pose it in the form of a serious question, namely: What management strategies and styles do staff consider are most appropriate to support more team-based NHS organisations and why? By phrasing it this way I am suggesting that the interplay between team behaviours, managerial psychology and organisational (corporate) cultures needs to be more fully understood. There is some important research that illuminates the problems with team working in more hierarchical organisations, outside healthcare (Prasad 2001), particularly in relation to difficulties about staff motivation, cooperation and their ability to act as coherent teams. Every team does not need the same kind of managerial support. What are perceived by staff to be more controlling, liberating, empowering management styles is closely linked to a team's ability to make decisions, be innovative and influential. I will return to these issues in Part Four.

A lived scenario: reflecting on inter-professional teams

'I was working as a social worker in a newly established inter-professional team, which was itself part of a research study, working to discharge stroke patients early from hospital, providing rehabilitation in patients'

own homes. The team had no opportunity for any team building activities, or discussions prior to taking referrals, and team members initially worked from different worksites. … it is important to identify and evaluate the positive characteristics of good inter-professional working. The aim of this research was therefore to try to analyse and evaluate these features in the team in which I worked' (Molyneux, 2001, pp. 29–30). This work was done through a semi-structured interview method, content analysis of the transcripts, feedback and reappraisal with team members. Two conclusions of this work are not surprising, but helpfully confirm:

- The team felt it worked well because of their personal qualities of flexibility and adaptability, which enabled them to move across conventional professional boundaries with confidence. This latter point was linked with Laidler's state of 'professional adulthood' (Laidler 1991) and Gilbert *et al.*'s (2000) work about the things that make inter-professional teams work well.
- Good communication was essential between members and particularly the way joint case notes both improved working relationships and helped members understand each other's roles. Team meetings and team briefings (Oliver & Tonks 1998) were significant opportunities for improving communication.
- The third conclusion was about a team's 'working frameworks'. Molyneux (2001, p. 340) writes, *'Articulating disciplinary and professional identity is important before inter-professional relationships can be successful. It is difficult to form collaborative ties when one is unsure of one's professional identity (Dombeck 1997, p. 15). Team members were able to achieve this, and as a result establish a team based on an egalitarian, co-operative approach to their work together, and in partnership with patients. Healthcare professionals need to reflect on, and reconsider their attitudes, approaches and expectations towards both traditional ways of working and professional power balances in inter-professional settings'.* The point here was that this was a newly formed team and this presented a particular opportunity for staff. There were no pre-existing guidelines or criteria for team working. No team history. They were making history. There can be problems when staff feel there is not a framework within which to work (Flory 1998). But this team turned it into an opportunity to invest in the creation of their own framework with all the attendant team learning benefits that can accrue from this. For example, the sharing of experience and expertise, a sense of ownership and therefore shared responsibility and accountability and an opportunity to show how creative they can be in meeting patients needs.

Reflecting on 'care-in-the-round' and wraparound teams

What is a view of a multi-professional, wraparound, reflective team, as a modern team for a modern twenty-first century NHS? We might simply describe it as wraparound because those that comprise the team, this may be healthcare professionals, administrative and support staff, social, welfare, justice, education, family, friends and so on, wrap themselves around the service user. It positions, or situates, the user in the centre of the action. This is both symbolic and practical. Symbolic in the sense that the team makes a statement of the kind, 'We believe the user should be the centre of our attention'. It can be read as a value statement. This conception of a modern team means that membership is flexible. It is not just who is part of the team but more what the team does and stands for.

This wraparound notion is supportive of the statement about the future nurse that we find in the Royal College of Nursing discussion paper *The Future Nurse* (RCN 2003, p. 11). In paragraph 10.3 they state, '*The paper has made reference to the importance of a patient-centred approach without clarification of why or what that might mean. The literature on patient-centred care defines it in terms of redesigning systems so that they meet patients' need for care-in-the-round rather than the organisational need to manage/monitor/categorise care*'. In a later paragraph (10.6) we find, '*There are some radical options to consider in this debate. If systems are designed around patients' need for care-in-the round, based on the concept of need for particular forms of care rather than categories of illness, the way in which healthcare systems are currently organised would have to change. If the quality of care is the primary objective rather than the category of disease/medical specialism, admission to a general surgical or ortho-paedic ward might change to a ward centred on rehabilitative care or women's health. . . . This would represent a radical change in thinking not only about how healthcare systems might be re-organised and re-categorised, but a fundamental re-think about what healthcare is and what within it benefits patients*' (RCN 2003, p. 12).

There is a strong suggestion here that 'normal' professionalism (Chambers 1998) needs to give way to 'new' professionalism. The former is characterised by the values and behaviours of the dominant in healthcare and by 'high-status' disciplines. This is about their power and knowledge generation, reproduction, management, transfer and application. New professionalism reverses the normal flows of knowledge, values and traditional patterns of power relations and puts front line staff and service user views first. But let's keep this in proportion. What I am advocating is keeping and sustaining what works, but also opening up the possibilities for dialogue about what might help to make services better. This opening up of possibilities is about considering new and better ways of team learning.

Normal professionalism is a mindset where teams are normally and overwhelmingly made up of healthcare professionals. Have you ever heard of a team of service users? Maybe not yet! Maybe they are still called focus, stakeholder or liaison groups? New professionalism is supported by documents like *Shifting the Balance of Power* (DoH 2002c) and *Managing for Excellence* (DoH 2002b). Looking at this optimistically, new conceptions of teams bring with them the hope for new epistemologies about and for practice. This is likely to involve having different and perhaps difficult kinds of conversation. The Royal College of Nursing's idea of care-in-the-round is a wonderful catalyst to get us to further clarify the role of human agency, new kinds of teams, those conceived as communities-of-learners and the closely associated notions of choice, accountability, responsibility and free will that go with this kind of possibility (Barnes 2000, Wenger 2002).

Teams as communities of learners

Central to questions about what makes teams work well is *team learning*. An underlying assumption is that good teams comprise good learners (Offenbeek 2001). The growing emphasis on team working, in the NHS, may well create gaps between working and learning. This is often symptomatic of 'busy-busy' cultures. All doing and no reflecting. Gaps between knowing and doing, between thinking and acting. We need more investment in looking at team learning processes, in action, in the workplace. Much can be learned from the excellent work being done in places like the University of Middlesex in England and Queens University in Belfast on workplace learning. Hopefully, the Institute for Innovation and Improvement will also play a key role in this. Team learning rests upon assumptions and understandings that we have about human behaviour and particularly about participation, about leadership, power, the expression of emotion, diversity, and about conflict, for example. It is a complex process in itself and embedded within workplace cultures. These can enable or inhibit learning. In certain workplaces, all learning may not be fun.

Much of the change-speak in the NHS is currently focused on a process of 'modernisation'. We find three components of this in the NHS Modernisation Agency's publication, *Improving Performance in the NHS* (DoH 2003). A modernising NHS means:

- *Renewal*. More modern buildings and facilities, new equipment and information technology, more and better trained staff
- *Redesign*. Services designed in radically different ways with a much greater use of clinical networks to better co-ordinate services around the patient.
- *Respect*. A culture of mutual respect between politicians and the NHS, between different groups of staff in the service and crucially, between the NHS and those we serve.

Due to this emphasis I wonder what teams might have to learn in order to sustain themselves through a modernisation process? Three suggestions are:

1   To develop a sense of one's place in a bigger picture of NHS reform.
    An understanding that others are going through what the team is
    going through right now.
2   To develop a strong sense of teamness, a team-as-a-community, learn-
    ing and growing together where relational ties are known and secure.
3   To develop a team culture of reflection where growth is through team
    learning from grounded experiences and empowering acts.

With regard to 1 above, teams can benefit if they are able to network
with others, where similar (and different) stories to their own are told
and reflected upon. This can help teams to feel more comfortable about
what's happening to them. The key here is to find nets-that-work, clinical
networks and more! With regard to **2**, feeling and expressing fears and
concerns requires a sense of safety, and compassionate and respectful
listening from others in the team. Again trust is an important part of this.
The key issue here is how far staff, who make up a particular team, feel
they have access to others they trust enough to express and to work
through difficult feelings and challenging issues. What I am alluding to
here is a view of a team as a *community-of-learners*.

Reflecting on team leaders

Leaders and (clinical and political) leadership are currently receiving
much attention, particularly through the Royal College of Nursing Leadership Project and their LEO Programme. Katzenbach & Smith (2003,
p. xviii) argue that '... the team leader is seldom the primary determin-
ant of team performance'. They also claim that the choice of leader is
significant and that the role is not always an easy one. A variety of people
and personalities can lead teams effectively. Debates about the need for
and nature of a team leader, have been stoked-up by the work of Beverly
and John Alimo-Metcalfe (2003). The background to this article was their
1998 study into stress levels in the NHS. It comprised a sample of 11 000
NHS staff. Their findings were 'very worrying'. In 1998 they concluded,
'Probably about 27% of NHS staff are minor psychiatric cases'. In 2003
they write, 'Five years on, who would seriously claim stress levels are
decreasing? This raises serious questions about the quality of leadership
in the NHS' (Alimo-Metcalfe & Alimo-Metcalfe J, 2003, p. 28). They go on
to pose the question: What really makes a good leader? In their conclusions they align the term 'NHS manager' with leader. The lowest scores
for managers, derived from their transformational leadership questionnaire (TLQ) show the (relative) areas of (leadership) weakness to be
associated with:

- inspiring others;
- supporting a developmental culture;
- showing genuine concern;

- encouraging change;
- being honest and consistent; and
- acting with integrity.

'Showing genuine concern' was found to be the single most important indicator of transformational leadership. 'Worryingly this is among the weakest dimensions of leadership in the NHS' (Alimo-Metcalfe & Alimo-Metcalfe 2003, p. 29). Perhaps it is time to re-think what we mean by a 'leader' and what leader*ship* is, especially in the context of our developing understandings of the nature of teams and how team membership is experienced? In Part Four I will be describing the qualities of '*quiet leaders*' and how they work to develop reflective teams.

The untapped potential of team performance is enormous in most NHS organisations. Well-meaning aspirations like 'we need to work better as a team' will barely be sufficient either to develop them or to overcome resistance to them. The 'right' team, in the 'right' place, at the 'right' time for the 'right' patient/s might be the difference between widespread team achievement or random team successes. At the Institute of Health Managers UK annual conference, 2002, Professor Michael West stressed that organisations with a high level of team working had significantly lower in-patient mortality rates than other organisations. He said that effective team working also had a marked impact on reducing stress levels among employees and reducing staff turnover. He suggested that the key lesson to be learned was that people who know what is expected of them and feel they are working in a supportive environment, are much more effective staff (Institute of Health Management 2002, p. 7).

Chapter 12

The centrality of values

Values are fundamental to everything we do. 'Identify your values. Come to know what you believe. Come to know what is most important to you. Come to recognise when your values are tested. Only when you can stand up to the test, are your values truly validated and confirmed' (Jones & Jones 1996, p. 13).

The value ... a commitment to care

It is reasonable to assume that those who work in and with the NHS have a commitment to care. It seems obvious in an everyday sense. In general, most human beings want to try to care for others and be cared for. *Caring* is a core value of the National Health Service. So why do we care about caring? Or phrased in a less philosophical way: What do members of a team mean when they say they care? Care means many things. Care can be linked with *cares*, which can be equated with burdens. 'I have lots of things on my plate, burdens, worries. I'm fretting over things'. It can be used in the sense of caring for someone. This may have something to do with a desire or inclination towards someone else, or maybe a regard for their views or their particular stand on things. This expression of care is caring about ideas. There is also caring about things. 'He only cares about the money.' 'She only seems to care about balancing her budget.' Imagine a situation where you find yourself having to care for an elderly family member. You may feel you have a responsibility for their physical and psychological wellbeing. Can you claim to care for this family member if what you do is perfunctory or grudging? Arguably caring for others and trying to be nice to colleagues is a good idea when trying to get things done. But we must always be mindful that there is something called the 'tyranny of niceness' (Street 1995). Being 'nice' can sometimes get in the way of getting things done, especially when this involves making tough decisions, a potential loss of face and time pressures.

Creating an enabling team context that encourages caring, cooperation, sharing, loyalty, creativity and participation sounds appealing, even though we again need to be mindful of the 'tyrannies of participation' (Hickey & Mohan 2004). The key thing is how do we get caring 'front and central' in the culture of teams? von Krogh *et al.* (2000) put forward five helpful dimensions of care, namely: mutual trust, active empathy, access to help, lenience of judgement and courage. These are important attributes of a team which I argue (in Part Four) contribute to a team's *wellness*.

- *Mutual trust.* In every encounter with another person we establish some degree of trust with them. We cannot know all their motives, preferences, interests, personal background, opinions of you, reactions to your conversations, backing in the organization, ability to follow-up agreements the two of you have made, and so forth.
- *Active empathy.* While trust creates the basis for caring, active empathy makes it possible to assess and understand what other members in the team truly need. Empathy is the attempt to put ourselves in the shoes of the other, understanding their particular situation, interests, skill level, success, failures, opportunities and problems. By active empathy, von Krogh *et al.* (2000) mean that we proactively seek to understand the other. We do this through active questioning and alert observations. Unfortunately, because there *are* numerous barriers to dealing with emotional issues in most organisations, expressing needs, especially emotional needs, can be difficult for staff.
- *Access to help.* Active empathy prepares the ground for helping behaviour, but care in the team has to extend to real and tangible support. The will to support others has to be accompanied by access to those who can provide help. What good is a manager who is never available to their staff? Additionally, what good are clinical leaders who protect themselves from junior staff because they are reluctant to give away their preciously acquired knowledge and skills? Under such circumstances, some staff may commit to the idea of care and helping, but in practice they do not make themselves available.
- *Lenience in judgement.* For care to be securely embedded in patterns of staff relationships, it has to be complemented with a lenient attitude amongst team members. Members have to learn to control their own judgemental impulses.
- *Courage.* Courage plays an important role in team development and wellness in three ways. First, staff must be courageous when expressing and trying out new ideas and practices, in the company of others. Second, staff need to be brave when doing this as they are expressing a commitment to something that may be open to challenge. Third, it takes courage to voice your opinion or give feedback as part of a process that helps other members grow. von Krogh *et al* (2000) argue that as feedback may be negative or disruptive for the individual, great courage is required by those who offer it, even if they are lenient judges.

A modernisation process puts particular demands on teams and member relationships. In order to really work as a team, members have to share personal knowledge. Others need to listen and react to what is being said. Caring, constructive and helpful relationships are required for this. Valuing care and team learning are inextricably linked. I acknowledge Mayeroff's (1971) view, which is presented in von Krogh *et al.* (2000, p. 47), namely, '... *to care for others is to help them learn; to increase their awareness of important events and conse-quences; to nurture their personal knowledge while sharing their insights'.* I will re-visit these dimensions of care in Part Four.

How far are values everywhere?

Values are everywhere, so I guess they matter. Mattering about them matters. Values are also multi-faceted and contentious. Values are so-cially constructed and need to be consciously and critically reflected upon. They need to be a central feature of team-talk and if necessary, modified over time and with experience. Carr (1992) says that values are much like principled preferences. He argues that these are of '... quite considerable importance' and that, 'unlike other sorts of preferences which are based merely on personal taste or natural disposition, values are standardly a consequence of something approaching intelligent de-liberation and are thus, in principle, susceptible of rational appraisal and re-appraisal' (Carr 1992, p. 244). For example, you may have a view with regard to the UK government's establishment of foundation trusts. This view is unlikely to be based upon a whim or fancy but more to do with a principled preference. By implication this makes us valuing beings and our work value-laden.

Values manifest themselves in things we read, like in a mission state-ment, and business and action plans. Sometimes we need go no further than the title of major government policy documents to get the feel for the values that might be espoused therein. Good examples of this are *Working Together – Learning Together* (DoH 2001a), *Liberating the Talents* (DoH 2002a), *Shifting the Balance of Power* (DoH 2002c) and *Improving Working Lives* (DoH 2002d). There are many values embedded in the Nursing and Midwifery Council's statement called, *Supporting Nurses and Midwives Through Lifelong Learning* (NMC 2002). These are values related to the nature of staff support and commitments to lifelong learning. When reading the Commission for Health Improvement's (2003) report on the NHS called, *Getting Better?* we not only read about what is valued by the Commission, namely, the experience of those who use the NHS. We are also led into the complex area of value judgements. These are gener-ated by the Commission's commitment to explore two serious questions. First: What do people want from the NHS? Second: What are the hallmarks of organisations that are improving?

Values can also be heard. For example, when Prime Minister Tony Blair took up office in May 1997, he espoused a commitment to 'decent values'. In general this commitment embraced notions of com-passion, social justice, liberty, fighting poverty and inequality, and so on

(Runnymede Bulletin 1997). The re-appointed Welsh health minister Jane Hunt spoke exclusively to the *Health Services Journal* (Betts 2003) and espoused a very clear value position, a Welsh health policy based on collaboration and partnership. 'We are a family which works closely together.' She went on to pledge herself to improve team working. It would be '... vital that local health boards learned how to work together, across boundaries' (Betts 2003, p. 9). We are hearing more and more sound bites from human resource people who market the complexities of the NHS in a phrase like the golden trust, the model employer, the skills escalator, the model career, and so on. Each sound bite is replete with values.

Values do not float around in some kind of void. Neither do they grow on trees or fall like manna from heaven. They do not even look after themselves. Values are located historically, socially, culturally and politically. They are embedded in what we say or choose not to say, in what we feel, do and do not do. So how might this discussion about values link with the notion of teams? Some argue that teams have a 'common' purpose, a common goal or way of doing things. The idea of things in 'common' is a way of expressing the essence of a team. They unify something that can be very diverse. So what actually is it that might unify this diversity? What might connect members together into a team and keep them behaving like one, under pressure? What enables them to have this common purpose? What provides the rationale, the reasons if you like, for feeling and doing one thing rather than another? What actually provides this commonality or what I prefer to call *connectedness*?

I am not simply speaking about connections that arise from doing the same things, in the same places, with the same service users. I am thinking not only of a connection of hands, but a connection of heads, hands and hearts (Wakhlu 1999). A connection of hearts amongst a group of healthcare staff brings with it the possibility of transforming them into a team. A connection where emotion, soul and spirit come together (Ghaye 2005). This gives a team, at the very least, an identity and integrity. By identity I mean feelings and experiences that make them who they are. By integrity I mean those feelings and shared experiences that are integral to our personhood. By including the word spirit I mean the many ways we might think about and act in relation to 'team spirit'. Something that animates our appreciation of each other and animates our work.

I am of course proposing here an optimistic view of values as things that help us connect and might enable us to feel part of a real team. Feelings associated with a sense of belonging, shared commitment and understandings. A collective sense of moral purpose and accountability. For some teams, these feelings may not be readily perceived and known through our physical senses. Feelings like courage, trust, goodness, forgiveness, kindness and joy. To this I would also add soul. 'It needs soul to see these qualities and in a cynical environment that destroys the soul, these qualities cannot be recognised. Courage is then seen as foolhardiness, truth as naivety, goodness is plain daft, beauty is completely irrelevant, forgiveness does not exist, patience is tested and fails, compassion is alien, kindness is soft-in-the-head, trust is foolishness and joy is not a word to be used' (Lamont 2002, p. 3).

However, values can also serve to disunite, disconnect and highlight difference. For some, difference and diversity are welcomed and fostered. But not by everyone. Professor Ian Kennedy's £14 million, 3-year inquiry, which examined the treatment of 1827 children who had heart surgery at the Bristol Royal Infirmary between 1984 and 1995, made reference to a 'club culture'. If you were in the club you were fine. If you were not it was difficult to raise concerns or be heard if you did raise them. National newspapers of the time carried headlines like, 'Conspiracy of silence behind the needless death of 35 infants' (Duckworth & Morris 2001). This is clearly a most dramatic example of a certain set of values that served to create a club culture with surgeons at the centre of it. So holding a value or values and living them out in practice should not be regarded as an easy, straightforward and rational thing.

This gives rise to two serious questions. First: *What values does a team hold?* Second: *Which values have (or appear to have) more legitimacy and authority?* By this I mean which values are more appropriate in which contexts? The first question is about what the team's values actually are. The second is a normative issue of what they should or might be. But these questions embrace another concern. It is to do with knowing how to reconcile the differences that we have in holding certain values rather than others. In the context of healthcare teams and their relationship with their organisation, it is a concern over knowing what to do when colleagues either do not appreciate, or wish to subscribe to, a particular value or values. What happens if we value self-determination, autonomy and independence, when other members in the team value collegiality, collaboration and working together? Can these apparently incompatible values be reconciled?

Values from elsewhere and from within

I have said that values are everywhere. They are 'out there' and from a distance. I would call this from 'elsewhere'. But they are also 'in here', from 'somewhere' close to us. This somewhere is inside us and the team. We need to reverse customary thinking that only acknowledges values from elsewhere. If a colleague is heard to exclaim 'Nobody cares!' what can we read into this? How far might it reflect a frustration with their increasing immersion in bureaucratic procedures, committees and piles of paperwork? When a colleague says, 'I've no choice but to leave and work somewhere else. I don't really feel I belong', what does this mean?

How far might this say something about legitimate decision-making, control and freedom, expectations, fears, hopes and so on? If a colleague says, 'I really think I'm hitting my head against a brick wall', what are they really saying? How far might this reflect a difference in value positions held, expressed and actioned? With regard to the articulation of team values we might usefully reflect on the following.

1   How might we come to know the more privately held values of our team members?
2   How far are we able to acknowledge and/or resolve any difficulties that may arise, within the team, from members holding a diversity of values?
3   What is the link between what we say (our espoused values) and what we do (our values-in-action)?
4   How far can we live out our values more fully in our practice?

Two serious questions that arise are: What organisational or other influences prevent me/us working in different ways? What alternatives are indeed available to us?

We often assume that values held, like those linked with a duty of care, are best understood in the relationships between the ones-caring and those cared-for. In the normal course of events, we might expect some kind of action from those who claim to care. The assumed relationships between values and practice need quite a lot of careful thought. Healthcare may be regarded as a collection of professions because the values espoused are professed in and through healthcare practices. A prime task for each healthcare team therefore is to work out what their values are, not in isolation and abstraction, but jointly with colleagues amidst the complexities of clinical and managerial life. We might usefully tackle these tasks with Goldhammer (1966, p. 49) in mind. '*The vast majority ... of values and assumptions from which our ... professional behaviour is governed are implicit. They're inarticulate, they're nebulous, they're buried someplace in our guts and they're not always very accessible ... We can't always rationalise exactly what we're doing ... We can't always make explicit the justifications for the acts we perpetrate ... Only after these things have been made explicit, have been brought to the point where you can enunciate the damn things, can we begin to value those that seem to have some ... Integrity and disregard those that seem to be inane.*'

Saying one thing and doing something else

This whole business of knowing, espousing and trying to live values through our actions, has been helpfully and provocatively explored by the many writings of Jack Whitehead from the University of Bath, UK (Whitehead 1993, 2000, Whitehead with Johns 2000) and with others in the context of educational action research (McNiff & Whitehead 2001,

2002). You may also find it helpful to consult Jack's website and explore his thoughtful and relevant idea of learning to live values of humanity more fully in practice and how this connects with 'living theory' (http://www.bath.ac.uk/~edsajw). These are challenging ideas and putting anything into practice and living through our values, might feel impossible some days! The complexity and importance of these ideas is illustrated through the scenario with Ruth and Peter.

A lived scenario: caring moments with Peter

This scenario portrays the connections between values, actions and the quality of a patient's life. Ruth writes about her encounter with one of her patients. His name was Peter. The encounter Ruth describes lasted approximately 90 minutes. Ruth worked as part of a hospice team. In this account Ruth is working as a nurse practitioner. Her job entailed seeing all elective patients prior to surgery to undertake a holistic assessment, to asses their nursing, medical, psychological, social and spiritual needs. What values do you discern in her practice?

> 'One morning, when taking the opportunity to prepare for a busy afternoon clinic by looking through the medical records of those patients booked in for pre-operative assessment; one of the staff nurses on the ward, ran into my office asking if I would go onto the ward as one of the patients was calling for me. The staff nurse appeared worried, so instantly stopping my work we hastened to the ward.
>
> There seemed a lot of commotion on the ward, the noise level was high, and the attention was drawn to the gentleman in the corner bed who was shouting my name loudly. Knowing him well, I went instantly to his side. Peter was very agitated and distressed, clinging to my hand he exclaimed, "I'm dying aren't I? Ruth you have always been straight with me, tell me the truth now, I'm dying aren't I" Sitting next to Peter, and taking both of his hands into mine while looking straight into his eyes, I spoke softly to try and calm and reassure him, saying, "I can feel your distress, and want to help you, but before we can address your fears let us try to make you feel a little calmer so that you can concentrate on what we discuss." While continuing to speak softly, Peter was asked to breathe slowly and deeply. I reminded him of our open and honest relationship, and reassured him that his questions would be answered with the same honesty.
>
> When Peter was calmer, the curtains around his bed were closed to ensure a little more privacy. Returning to my seated position facing Peter, and holding his hands in mine whilst maintaining eye contact, I asked him what had caused his distress. He responded by saying that he had an overwhelming feeling that he was going to die imminently and that he wanted someone to tell him honestly if this was going to happen. My response was, "Peter, what do you know about your illness?" He said, "I know I've got cancer and that it has

spread into other parts of my body." I confirmed that this was true and that this meant he was very ill. He then said, "It is going to kill me isn't it?" My reply was, "Yes Peter, the cancer will probably cause you to die, but before that, you have a lot of living to do." He responded, "What do you mean?" "You are seriously ill with advanced metastatic cancer and you are very weak, but you have a wonderful family and you have told me you want to spend more time with them. Having a lot of living to do, means that you should spend this stage in your life living and doing those things which are most important to you. Talk to your family; say the things you want to say and do the things you want to do. Make every moment special, live life with the cancer, rather than die with the cancer."

With these words Peter cried silently, then squeezed my hands. He then asked me to call his wife. He wanted to see her and tell her that he loved her. Peter insisted on my staying with him while his wife came to the ward. He held my hand firmly and whispered, "please don't leave". Speaking softly and calmly to Peter talking about all of the wonderful things that he had told me about his wife and children, concentrating on the laughter, love and the fun they shared together, he began to smile. When his wife arrived on the ward Peter was calmer and they held onto each other both silently crying. When attempting to leave, Peter asked if I could stay a while, he said "I still need some of your strength." He then turned to his wife and said, "I feel more in control now, I know I'm going to die, but it will be when I am ready. I need to spend more time with you and the boys first; Ruth has helped me see that. I love you, and want to tell you, I want you to remember that when I am gone." They held each other again and, although tears, there was also a great sense of happiness. Peter soon relaxed back into his pillows exhausted with emotion, he squeezed my hand and said, "You can go now. Thank you for your help; you have given me back my life."

On leaving the room, my own feelings and tears surfaced, a feeling that I had done so little, but glad that it was helpful if only in a small way. Peter died in his wife's arms two weeks later, after saying his goodbyes to all his family and friends. At Peter's funeral his wife hugged me, and thanked me for helping them, saying that I was in the right profession."

Ruth conveyed to me that a move to a hospice environment enabled her to come to know what she describes as the essential attributes of patient care. She summarises these as follows. She calls it a statement of intent and of value. It is something she keeps with her and tries to live out in her work.

'I feel that a patient should be enabled to live until they die, at their own maximum potential, performing to the limit of their physical activity and mental capacity, with control and independence wherever possible. They should be recognised as the unique person they are and helped to live as part of their family (however this might be defined) and in other relationships with some awareness from those around of their own hopes and expectations and of what has deepest meaning for him.'

See Hardie (2000) for a full version of Ruth's reflections.

One point of personal growth for Ruth was to move forward with this statement of 'intent and value' and explore its connectedness with the statements of others, tacitly or explicitly known by staff, in her working environment. But making values more known is easier said than done. For each member of a team it is important that any values that become regarded as 'our values' are freely chosen. What values become team values need to be chosen from an array of alternative ones. In deciding what values will reflect what the team stands for, each member needs to think about and articulate the consequences of holding these values. Potentially more problematic is the degree of congruence between the values held by a team and those of their organisation. This potential tension can be related to recruitment, retention and return to work issues so prevalent in the NHS. Sometimes staff feel that they only have three options when there is a mal-alignment regarding values. You put up and shut up. You leave and go to work somewhere else, or you do something about these differences! What option is chosen might depend upon the nature of the differences between us and the support we feel we might get, from others, if we tackle them.

Values and actions ... some concerns

There are at least six potential kinds of value-related concerns. They are not mutually exclusive. They are concerns to do with value:

1 Blindness.
2 Confusion.
3 Tokenism.
4 Conquest.
5 Alienation.
6 Conflict.

Teams need to be appreciative of the potential for enablement and corrosion that each concern brings with it. For most teams it tests their collective ability to make, what they may perceive to be 'problems', their friends.

Value blindness

In conversations with teams about their values, I often find myself engaging with conversations that may contain the concerns expressed by Kate,

> 'Yes I know, we do have values ... of course we do, we have to... and especially given what we do ... even though we may not call them this. We know they're there, well around somewhere anyway. But this is the first time we have been asked, formally like this, to talk about them ... like this, all

together… Maybe we just assume we have the same values? They are a bit personal really. I agree we need to be aware of them… how we put words to them is hard though isn't it? I would think we could be in for a lively discussion!'

(with thanks to Kate, Senior Charge Nurse, HIV and Sexual Health Team in a Primary Care Trust).

The concerns raised here by Kate are alluding to *value blindness*. We know we have reasons for doing what we do. We may not be fully aware of them. We may not call them values. We know that in caring, the values of the one-caring, may be seen in her/his acts of caring. But the action component, the link between caring-and-acting is problematic. More specifically and directly, if we hold values of care they carry with them a commitment to some action in relation to the cared-for. The problematics centre on the business of observable action and how caring is conveyed to the cared-for. Sometimes we hear reference to the trilogy that we should be able to *describe, explain* and *justify* our practice. In description we need to select what it is we want to describe, in what ways and for what reasons. In explanation we need to think about how we are actually able to do this! What do we appeal to, what standards, criteria and the like? What frames of reference? We know that merely saying, 'I attended to this patient in this way because that's the way I've always done it', does not cut the mustard. And then there is the issue of justification. Our values can offer us justifications for our practice, reasons for doing things.

Developing teams brings with it a need to make that which is personally known (Polanyi 1958), more explicit, publicly available for discussion and exploration. There are a range of methods that help make the tacit more explicit within teams. Some are paper-and-pencil activities, some more expressive ones (Parkinson 1997, Hunt & Sampson 1998, Novak 1998, Ghaye & Lillyman 2001, Higgs & Titchen 2001, Kember et al. 2001). Making the tacit more explicit might include the use of painting, dance, music, photography, drama, mod-roc modelling, and so on. Each approach brings with it certain risks. Safety is often a personal thing, not easily determined by another. Each can carry with it the possibility of making the private a little more public. For example, a team of six critical care nurses were all feeling buffeted by the winds of change in the NHS. They felt they were losing 'something' but they were not sure what this 'something' was. Work was just beginning to feel different. Some felt there was 'more tension in the air'. Others said that 'It seems harder and harder to do what I'm here for'. One member said that she felt they were being 'torn apart'. But collectively they felt they had the courage, not to wait any longer, but to try to confront some of these feelings. They worked together for 5 days spread over 15 weeks.

After the first couple of meetings it was clear to everyone that each member of the team had a different contribution to make to the conversation. Staff had to work with issues about what they were going to trust each other with. Perhaps just as significant was that each member of the team had their own preferred learning style. At the end of the first session three things emerged. First, staff did not want to 'just sit and talk about things'. Second, they wanted to bring together, in some way, what they all thought about their working lives on the unit. Third, they expressed a need to ' . . . *have a record of what we do, to reflect on in the future*'. A decision was made. Staff would jointly resource a practical activity that they would do together. When they felt they had gone as far as they could with it, they agreed to write something about their 'creation'. This was a large collage, 3 × 4 feet, as shown below.

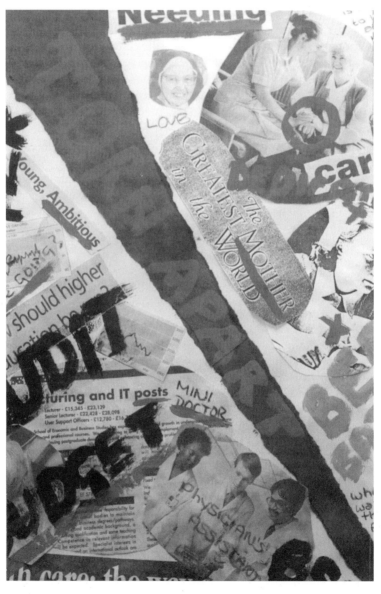

Fig 12.1   Learning to see: a staff collage.

A lived scenario: value blindness

'We all brought in some newspapers, magazines and brochures about the NHS, nursing and so on, that we agreed to do from last time. With some sense of excitement and a little trepidation we made a start. We each had a piece of paper and tried to express some of our feelings and moods, about our work, by using a simple pencil. Fine lines depicted soft, warm and gentle feelings, to dark thick lines expressing boldness or aggression. We had some views on how to use flowing lines increasing and decreasing in intensity to show mood shifts or different feelings. We then began to explore working with pictures and words that we had brought in. We cut out words and pictures that meant something special to us and others that represented some of those things that we felt might be affecting our work on the unit and our feelings of working together as a team. We looked at what each of us had done, moved words and pictures between us, talked about them, discarded some, laughed about and became very focused on others. We then took some blank white paper, black and grey pieces of card, stencils, black and white paint and charcoal sticks. And then the crunch. We tried to create a collage which expressed something of our collective feelings about 'Us as a team of critical care nurses, in the place where we work.' We tried to sustain an on-going conversation, between us, as we immersed ourselves in creating our collage. This wasn't hard as we wanted to make the collage represent a clear image of how we were feeling, right now. What was interesting was all the talk about the things we cared most about and what we thought was getting in the way. We didn't all agree, all of the time. But what we did agree on was that if we wanted to say something, we would be listened to by all the others.

With the materials we explored how we might create sharp, dramatic lines, zigzags, triangles and so on that might say more than words might. We used the paint in a bold way, over-writing other things with it. There was such a feeling of relief when we finally agreed to put 'torn apart' across the centre of our collage. We had finally been able to name it and talk about what it meant to each of us. The creation of our collage then seemed to be so much more meaningful. We felt it was a process of shared learning about what was tearing us apart, as we had been a very close team? We were dedicated to our work. We cared for our patients. But then there are 'all the other things to do', all in the name of progress and the way ahead. You can see this on our work. We feel this is really going to help us move on. We're hopeful anyway. What we felt as individuals is (mostly) on our collage ... we've got it out. Not easy but we felt it was rewarding. We feel it's brought us closer together. What we were blind to, we can now see a bit more clearly. And so to the next time. Where next now?'

(With thanks to the Critical Care Nurse Team in conversation with Tony, 5 November 2002.)

Value confusion

A second concern and a very common one, is *value confusion*. This often arises from having a long list of values. Sometimes 'the more the merrier' is a recipe for confusion. A list emerges and consensus rules OK. Nothing wrong with consensus of course as long as it is a genuine consensus and not one that is forced upon a team due to time constraints or other pressures from outside. It is sometimes hard to know what is and is not a value. 'Isn't everything we care about a value?' Some of the contents on these lists may be represented by a single word. Other parts of the list might contain lengthy phrases and statements of 'good intent'. It is wise to give conversations about clarifying confusion, time. Teams need to be patient with their own learning. Values need to be given a chance to bubble to the surface.

For example, some newly formed community mental health teams were given an opportunity to explore their views, hopes, anxieties, needs and wants in relation to the serious question: What do you feel will make your community mental health team, a team? Over a period of time, gently, patiently, each team in different ways engaged with this question. In the context of a conversation about the team's values (often referred to as 'the things we feel are really important to us') one team of nine staff made a list of 14 values they felt were necessary to become a team (see Table 12.1).

What is important is not whether they may be regarded as values or not, but the fact that a newly formed team engaged with this serious question. Behind lists like this lie many hopes, agendas and actions. Each word or phrase represents a multiplicity of meanings and this is a potential source of confusion. Some of them are to do with a need for intimacy and affiliation. Others to do with achievement and so on. What a list like this might mean to other teams, or the organisation, is another potential source of confusion. But an important start has been made.

Table 12.1   List of values.

Openness	Consistency of behaviour
Honesty	Mutual confidence
Fairness	Dependable
Keep promises to each other	Be competent
Loyalty	Being available and accessible
Meet our targets	Being seen to provide a good service
Respect each other's views	Learn from each other

Value tokenism

This is the practice of teams, who are only able at that time to make no more than a token effort or gesture in the direction of addressing the centrality of values in their practice. Another expression of tokenism is about making statements that we claim to be team values, actually writing them down, and then thinking 'job done'. This tokenism may be fleeting or a more subtle or sustained act of avoidance. Avoiding the implications they have for our sense of identity and self-worth. Tokenism can happen for a variety of reasons. Sometimes it happens when teams see the process of values clarification as 'just another task and the thing that teams have to do'.

A newly formed intermediate care 'team' of 30 staff confronted value tokenism. More accurately they were a group of 30 talented, passionate and experienced people, not a team. The interesting thing was that the group was made up of a number of unequal sized teams and one social worker who felt 'left out'. The situation was one of teams-within-a-group, a group comprising nursing, allied health and social care staff, qualified, unqualified, administrative and clerical staff. Due to a local process of re-organisation, a number of smaller 'teams', like a rapid response team, now found themselves 'in with others'. Each team had its own personalities, some 'big' ones, a sense of identity and a particular agenda. They also had histories. By this I mean a shared history of their own ways of doing things and with particular service users. They had stories to tell. But would others want to hear them? Would they understand them? Could they learn from them? The manager had created an opportunity for the group to come together for one afternoon, once every 3 to 4 weeks. The whole process lasted for 6 months. Her belief was that her staff needed some time to gel together as a new intermediate care team.

A lived scenario: value tokenism

Meeting One

Twenty two staff attended the first meeting. Most of the time was spent, with the manager present, exploring how the group might best use the space that had been created for them. The group had been on a 'vision day' three weeks prior to their first meeting. It was thought that this could be something that might be built upon. What soon became apparent was that although some proudly said, 'we've got our vision', this vision was not a collective one. Neither was it understood in the same way by members of the group. Perhaps a double whammy! After some animated discussion, staff collectively agreed to try to think again about the recurring themes in their conversation. They managed to turn these themes into three questions which some staff felt would be more 'real and concrete, to talk about and not more airy-fairy stuff'. These were:

- *What does the word team mean?*
- *What is an important thing I feel I could contribute to this newly formed intermediate care team?*
- *What is an important thing I feel I want from being part of this new team? (some interpreted 'want' for 'need')*

Staff agreed to think about these questions and to come back next time to explore them further.

Meeting Two

Twenty-five staff attended the second meeting. They used large and small pieces of coloured paper of different shapes, hoops and paper frames to see how far personal statements might find a friend in another person's statement, and sticky stars and arrows to try to illuminate connections between what was emerging. This was done in a large room, on the carpet, tables and the walls. All seemed to be going quite well. They appeared to be travelling fast, maybe too fast. Six statements kept coming round and around. Everything started to coalesce around them. Staff began to attach their personal statements to them. There was a growing feeling in the room that, 'yes, these were the things'. But were they the things that really represented their thoughts and feelings, or were they things they thought teams should have on their 'shopping list?' The six statements were 'being supported and supportive of each other', 'working together', 'respecting each other', 'trusting each other', 'feeling valued' and 'good communication including listening and honesty with each other'. These emerged as a list that was given a title, 'The key ingredients for our Intermediate Care Team'. They could also be read as an embryonic set of team values perhaps. Staff wrote each of these down on six large pieces of A1-sized paper. Before they departed they managed to agree that they would look more closely at one of the statements next time. The one chosen by the group was 'working together'. Inside this were two central issues. The need for a greater understanding of the different skills within the new group and how to get the best from this mix.

Meeting Three

The third meeting was also well attended. All the statements were placed in the centre of the floor. Before staff had completed their greetings someone asked, 'Who is going to be our team leader then, does anyone know?' This lit a fuse. The next hour was like a firework display. More exactly it was a very adversarial conversation between members of each of the teams that made up the group. A war-like tribal encounter. A question which opened up resentments, re-kindled memories of hopes that had been dashed in the past, provided opportunities for some staff to assert and position themselves in a particular way to others. Some presented mini c.v.'s, others began to describe the experience someone might need for the job. They talked over each other. Words like naïve, selfish, controlling, irrational and defensive were being used. There was conflict within and between people. There was also much arguing, which inhibited their ability to learn how others saw this issue. When they argued they traded conclusions. Throughout, their statements on the six large A1-sized pieces of paper, were on the floor, staring up at them. They were, at this point, merely tokens. They were not helping them to work together across and with differences. They needed to rescue themselves. They had to shift to a learning stance.

Value conquest, alienation and conflict

Value conquest is where one value, or set of values, effectively makes some staff passively and reluctantly surrender their value/s. This process is closely related to issues of power within the team. *Value alienation* is a more aggressive kind of problem for a team to work through. It is where values begin to be articulated, by some, which run counter to strongly held personal values. Common sources of this kind of alienation are, for example, related to problems over time attending to patients and 'doing all the paperwork', between standards of care and resources for this care, between a focus on patient through-flow and patient need, and so on. The final value related concern is *value conflict*. This can be a nasty team virus, eroding and undermining all those things that make a team, a team. Value conflicts can be to do with clashes, *impasse*, getting and staying stuck. For example one member passionately believes that patients should be fully involved and consulted in all aspects of their care because everyone has the fundamental right to self-determination. Other members take issue with this and the conflict shows in their actions. For example, operations are hastily explained to patients, parents and family with diagrams drawn on scraps of paper. The impression being given is one that informing patients and significant others, gaining their consent to treatment, is something of a chore.

Another example of value conflict might be to do with those members who actively wish to promote patient choice, with dignity and justice in mind, and those who hold other views. Perhaps those who do not wish to celebrate choice uncritically. The value position of promoting patient choice is tightly linked to patient empowerment and related issues like the patient as expert. Empowerment is a slippery, often misunderstood and much abused idea. There are many views of it. Conflicts may arise if team members do not fully appreciate this.

It is important that the view/s of empowerment a team uses are known and appreciated by all members. Conflicts can arise over issues to do with who actually becomes empowered. A team's conversation might not be about how much patients are empowered, but empowered for what reasons? There may be more conflict when values, that are linked with patient choice, get tangled up with manipulation, decoration (what teams and organisations look like rather than what they actually do) and tokenism. This is where some staff might feel choice becomes an empty ritual. Some members might be advocating choice passionately and stridently. Others may not see patient choice as a salvation narrative. Other members might be linking the discussion to related values such as equity. Serious questions like, 'How far will more choice mean better care for patients?' and 'How far will this mean equal treatment of those in equal need?' might be raised. These are tough questions and potentially fuel further conflict. But conflict is not always something that has, at all costs, to be avoided. Consensus is not the only way forward. Contrived consensus can, for some teams, be at least as problematic as certain forms of conflict.

Choice is not good just because it is choice, but because it is a way of affirming patient dignity and a commitment to social justice. By dignity I mean the recognition of who they are and respect for what they are. The

UK's Choice Agenda is part of a 'politics of participation' from a government that has championed partnership working since 1997. Choice is tied up in a general agenda of more service user activism. It can be seen as part of a (genuine) shift in the balance of power. We should avoid simplistic dichotomies when discussing the value of choice. We need to be mindful not to create moralistic dualities between participation and non-participation, having or not having choices. The promotion of patient choice needs to be a matter of personal and team reflection. 'Where do you stand if you, yourself, are not marginalised, excluded from or denied choice of services?' Perhaps if we feel 'this is me', we need to reflect upon the nature of our commitment to promoting patient choice?

Teams need to invest time in knowing 'what they stand for'. How we think about and care for all service users reflects who we are, what we believe in and stand for. When I say I care for a patient in rehabilitation resulting from a serious road accident, I am aware that I disclose something of my spirit and soul to them, my love of my discipline and a view of 'alongsideness'. Knowing oneself and knowing ourselves as team members, who we are and what we stand for, is as crucial to good healthcare practice as knowing our patients and our discipline. In fact if we do not know and cannot care for ourselves, how can we claim to know and care for others? If we do not know ourselves, how can we claim to know our subject, discipline, field or speciality in terms of deep, personal meaning? We may only know it abstractly, as 'stuff out there'. In other words as a commodity.

Chapter 13

Reflecting on the roles and contributions of the individual vis-à-vis the team

Scholtes *et al.* (1996) argue that a team out-performs individuals when:

- the task is complex;
- creativity is needed;
- the path forward is unclear;
- more efficient use of resources is required;
- fast learning is necessary; and
- high commitment is desirable.

This implies a shift away from cultures of individualism towards a greater focus upon learning and working competently together in teams. There are many sources of reference to this shift currently available (DoH 1997, 1998, 1999, 2000, 2001a, 2001b, 2002a, 2002b, 2002c, 2002d, 2003, NHS Modernisation Agency 2003).

What do we mean by working together?

A reference to this shift is described in Working Together-Learning Together (DoH 2001a), with many of its principles embraced in *Working Together: Staff Involvement, A self-assessment tool* (DoH 2000). The tool aims to help staff assess how much progress they feel their organisation has made in involving staff in planning as well as delivering services. The idea is that it is used in a joint review of progress by management and trade unions working in partnership. 'It is intended as a developmental process where the aim is to improve continuously, whether you are starting from a high or low level of partnership and involvement' (DoH 2000, p. 1). Progress is measured against seven standards (DoH 2000, p.2).

1 **Leaders** (including clinical leaders, union leaders, etc.) are committed to, and demonstrate, an involving culture.
2 People at all levels across the organisation understand and have the opportunity to influence its overall **vision and goals**.
3 There are **communication** processes up, down and across the organisation, which everyone understands clearly and can access readily.
4 There is a culture of **openness** in which staff feel free to contribute these ideas and voice concerns without fear or victimisation.
5 Responsibility is devolved to individuals and **teams** who can influence decisions about their work and working lives.

6   **Staff and trade unions** are effectively engaged at the earliest possible
    stage in influencing decisions and in joint information sharing, learn-
    ing and problem-solving with management.
7   All staff feel valued and are involved and supported in **developing**
    their knowledge, skills and potential.

What is interesting are the words and phrases that are highlighted (see
above) in the document. What is more significant are those that are not
highlighted. Two stand out particularly and will be elaborated upon in
Part Four. The first is the word *culture* which is explicitly mentioned in
two of the statements. Two descriptions of culture are given. An involving culture and a culture of openness. The other is the word *influence*,
which appears in three statements. In Part Four I will argue that shifting
from individualism to teams (standard 5) and the language of working
together and involvement, might most usefully be regarded as a culture
shift. This should not be downplayed. Consultations, committees, briefings, forums, team meetings, joint working parties, training events, sha-
dowing, job-sharing, participation in learning sets, and so on, under the
mantra of working together, is a discourse that not only shapes and
directs organisational behaviours but also helps to shape and inform
staff identities.

This self-assessment tool represents 'toolkit-talk'. Who actually makes
the assessment, be that an individual or a team, is a matter for debate. Who
is better placed to make judgements about working together? This kind of
talk is fast becoming a loud voice in the NHS. There are many toolkits
around and so lots of toolkit-talk. For example, the General Medical
Council and Department of Health's joint initiative has produced a toolkit
for general practitioners (GPs) and NHS consultants. There is also an
interesting toolkit for improving practice for general practices (Greco &
Carter 2002). We find many interesting examples of toolkits in the UK
government's recent initiative to modernise medical careers. Central to
this is a 2-year foundation programme of general training intended to form
a better bridge between medical school and specialist/general practice
training. Associated with this is, for example, a mini-PAT (peer assessment tool), a mini-CEX (clinical evaluation exercise) and DOPS (direct
observation of clinical skills). Other toolkits can be found through the
websites of the NHS Modernisation Agency and National Primary and
Care Trust (NatPaCT). What is important is the way toolkit-talk becomes
part of team-talk and nourishes cultures of working together.

What are we learning about individualism and cultures of separation that run counter to team cultures?

If cultures work against you, can you ever hope to get anything done? If
cultures clash and are antagonistic towards each other, can we ever think

of partnership working. If the dominant workplace culture is *'I come to work, get my head down, do my job and then go home again'*, what is the chance of team building and shared learning? Rather sadly a member of staff recently said to me, *'Working together. That's a joke. All we do is sit on opposite sides of the room and fire bullets at each other all day'*. She was referring to a joint working initiative between health and social care. But habitual patterns of work that promote individualism and cultures of separation seem to be slowly giving way to cultures of connection and integration. This will take time. For some staff working within, and even serving to promote, cultures of separation, it can be understood as a learned behaviour and an adaptive strategy. In doing this staff feel they can meet the most immediate demands on their time and expertise. Cultures of separation can promote feelings of privacy, even superiority and safety. This latter point is particularly the case in an NHS context of modernisation and reform in which the only privacy and safety some staff feel is left, the only place where they can be themselves, is in their own 'box'.

Another form of NHS culture is *balkanisation*. It can be prevalent in organisations where staff identify strongly with a discipline or perhaps work closely within a functioning unit. It is often expressed in loyalty to a group or team, rather than something bigger like a department, directorate or the organisation as a whole. Balkanisation is where groups and teams compete for scarce resources, status and influence in the organisation. *'If it serves the interests of "our team" then we will collaborate. If it doesn't then we see no need to.'* Some of the counter-currents here are those associated with more integrated care, multi-disciplinary, cross-boundary and multi-agency working. An involving culture and a culture of openness, mentioned earlier, focuses attention on what staff want 'working together' to actually mean. Is it to be perceived as a proper, patient-centred developmental process? How can staff avoid working together being perceived as a matter of coercion, compulsion and competition?

Working in more team-based learning cultures takes time to become a habit. Working supportively with others can be difficult when staff do not know much about who they are supposed to be supporting and why. If formal meetings are the only way staff can learn together and they find that meetings simply lead to more meetings, then what is the impact of this on their levels of interest and motivation? If having to stop, question current arrangements for working together and do things differently, is going to take an enormous effort, where is the energy and inspiration to come from? If doing necessary paperwork consumes important time needed to be spent in face-to-face contact with others in the team, then how might we do things differently? If protecting 'our interests' and our bit of turf, whatever this may be, is what we feel our job to be, then what does this say about learning and working together in teams?

Chapter 14

Reflecting on knowledge for competent practice

There has been a great deal written about knowledge for healthcare practice (Barbour 1995, Mallik *et al.* 1998, Rolfe & Fulbrook 1998, Johns 2002). Where it comes from, how useful it is regarded to be, how it might be transferred, applied, managed, and so on. The UK Royal College of Nursing has a useful website on the process of knowledge utilisation and transfer (www.rcn-ku.org.uk). Questions about knowledge are often a source of tension and confusion. Part of this is because there are so many views on the issue and so many ways of labelling knowledge. There are different kinds of knowledge. We might call them 'knowledges', a bit clumsy but true.

What is the importance of knowledge sharing and knowledge interaction in team development?

In collecting data for this book, I found that those staff who learned and shared wanted to learn more because they saw benefits to themselves, their team and their patients/clients. Learning and sharing to improve services is essentially about *knowledge management* and *knowledge interaction*. These are hot topics in the NHS! They are increasingly aligning themselves with discourses about and the practices of team development. For example, the Rapid Response Unit (RRU) of the NHS Clinical Governance Support Team was set up in 2002 to support 'nil star' and other 'challenged' NHS organisations. In the work they do with trusts, in health and social care and with strategic health authorities, they have adopted 'the BP model' (Collison & Parcell 2001) of knowledge management.
  McIntyre (2003, p. 10) states:

'At its core, knowledge management is about people. It is about how they behave and how they interact. It is about bringing together experiences of those who have the knowledge and those who need to know, at the right time and in such a way that relevant experience can flow throughout the organisation to where it is needed. Knowledge management also seeks to systematically liberate the richness of experience that is locked up in the mind of every individual within the organisation – the tacit knowledge – and to apply it to the organisation's goals. In other words to convert personal knowledge into organisational knowledge. The outcome of applying it successfully is better decision making, faster progress and a more cohesive and effect-ive organisation.'

There are two very interesting points made in this short article, which are highly relevant to this book. First, there is an acknow-ledgement that knowledge will not be shared if team (and organisational) cultures are not supportive of this. In cultures of separation and balkanisation, knowledge sharing is hugely problematic. Second, he talks about another kind of culture, one that is 'knowledge-centred' and which is open and inclusive. McIntyre very helpfully describes six attributes of such cultures. I present them below and then briefly respond to each one. McIntyre claims that knowledge-centred cultures are about:

- *Respecting people as individuals, which enables them to engage in valuable learning relationships.* I would argue that it is the team that is the crucible for learning now and in the foreseeable future.
- *Behaving in an open and inclusive manner, valuing the input of the wider team into specific goals.* Both openness and inclusivity are outcomes dependent upon other things like, what the team understands and experiences when they talk in terms of honest, frank, confidential and truthful inputs.
- *Practising communication skills and taking time to listen.* Communication is an extended family of skills. With some teams, practice not only needs to make perfect, but practice needs to make permanent as well. The time to listen to each other is a crucial ingredient to developing a sense of teamness.
- *Encouraging individuals to seek help and advice with issues.* A team provides a ready resource of potential help and advice. Who seeks advice and gets it, who seeks help, does not receive it and why, are all part of a knowledge sharing culture.
- *Identifying barriers to knowledge sharing and removing them.* Sometimes identifying the former is a little more easy than the actions of the latter! Much might depend upon the relationships between know-ledge and power that are influencing actions.
- *Relationships of trust and respect so that lessons may be shared, from failures to successes.* Trust is fundamental to knowledge sharing. But again there are complexities associated with this.

What is useful in the BP model is their process of 'peer assists'. This is all about getting staff talking. McIntyre describes this as a process that requires, '... *people to support each other; dedicating time to articulate and share information and insights; reflecting on what is known already prior to further engagement and using this pooled knowledge to decide what actions are possible*' (McIntyre 2003, p. 11). The RRU couple this with 'after action reviews' and a 'learning after' strategy. In another linguistic register these are the processes of reflection-on-action.

What knowledge matters most to team members?

Some might argue that the most important knowledge healthcare professionals need in order to do good work is a knowledge of how those they are caring for, those that are using healthcare services, are perceiving and experiencing their actions. This raises two serious questions. First, What matters most? Second, To whom? The issue is richly articulated by Clare, a gynaecology-oncology nurse practitioner working in a general hospital, in conversation with me.

> 'What I value most is a real understanding, knowledge if you like, of what is happening to my... well our patients. Without this all the skills I might have... or say I have anyway... don't mean much. All the skills in the world are irrelevant. I know how to look stuff up on the computer, do audits and the like. I also think I can have lively conversations with other staff on the ward... but without knowing what's going on inside the heads of my patients... how they are feeling, what they are thinking, needing and so on, I don't have a really good way of knowing what I could do that would be in their best interests. I know I can't ever really get inside my patient's mind... so to speak... you know what I mean... trying to experience what its like to be here as they experience it... am I making any sense? What I'm trying to say is I need to know this, or at least to try to get to know this. Of course there are risks... sometimes its better not to know. Sometimes when I find out things about them or their situation, say at home or with their family, things get complicated. Some things make me very proud of them... you know about their lives, the hardships they've had, their troubles... and now this. Knowing other things makes me realise that they have preferences and knowing this might mean that I have to change how I care for them... well at least reflect on how I am with them. I'm not saying that this is always a problem... what I mean is that I do value knowing this, but knowing this doesn't mean that everything suddenly becomes clearer... in fact sometimes it just adds to my sense of frustration and confusion. I think knowing how my patients are feeling and thinking about the care we are giving them, is the single most important thing. Knowing this can help to put us at our ease... but it can embarrass us. I'm being really honest now... we talk about this... as a team... what I think we all appreciate is that this kind of knowledge gives us a way of seeing what we do through the eyes of our patients. Sometimes what we think are quite small things... well not small but routine things... you know like greeting our patients, meal times, washing, doing the telly or getting some magazines, are hugely significant for them. We wouldn't know this if we didn't value trying to know this. Does any of this make sense?'

(With thanks to Clare in conversation with Tony, 9 June 2003.)

Schön (1991) also raised the serious question: What knowledge do practitioners need to know? He goes on to say that for him, it would be knowledge derived from '... reflections on the understandings already built into the skilful actions of everyday practice' (Schön 1991, p. 5). In this book I suggest that the question is expanded and put differently. We should appreciate that the knowledge practitioners need to know has at least three mutually supportive parts. First, there is knowledge for and about practice. Second, there is knowledge for and about public policy. Third, both of these kinds of knowledge come from within the team and from outside. All these kinds of knowledge guide what a healthcare team does and gives its members a sense of worth and identity. In reality, alas, things are not as clear cut as this. But this might be a helpful way of, at least, beginning to clarify our thinking about knowledge (or epistemological) issues. Knowledges for and about practice and policy are matters of negotiation, contestation and struggle between different individuals, groups and disciplines within health and other human service professions (Phillips 2000).

If the bottom line is that knowledge in healthcare needs to be useful and relevant, then we need to be sure what we mean when we employ these terms. Whatever knowledges a team generates and uses, they should all be a matter of scrutiny. Another serious question now arises, of the kind: In whose interests and for what purposes should this scrutiny be done? This debate is opened up when we posit a view of the practices of reflection as something that might usefully be regarded as intentional action leading to the possibility of improving services. Additionally, the role of reflexivity in the development of team knowledge should not be underestimated. This is where each team member engages in self-aware analysis of their own contribution to the team and the service/s it delivers. It is an awareness of how knowledge for better practice is co-constructed. This process of reflexivity was once linked closely with introspection and 'confessional tales' (Bleakley 2000). Now it might be regarded as an important source of team knowledge. The issue is to try to turn personal experience into more public and accountable knowledge for better services. The word 'better' will always be problematic (Griffiths 1998). What I am expressing is the need to reflect on the kinds of knowledge we need to learn, to use wisely and to good purpose.

Has knowledge a shelf-life?

Teams come and go. Teams are set up for particular reasons and then outlive their usefulness. Sometimes what they have done becomes part of an important history. It is valued by others that come after them. Sometimes it is forgotten because it is not regarded as important or relevant any more. Sometimes other teams learn from the work of earlier ones so there is a progressive development of what teams do and stand for. Sometimes the future is so uncertain that it is not possible to know what kinds of working arrangements (team-based or other) will be needed. You could substitute every reference that I have made to team with the word knowledge. For example, 'knowledge comes and goes'. Knowledge, is used for certain reasons then can out-live its usefulness. It gets dated, outmoded, over-taken by new knowledge. I take the view that it is wise to consider all knowledge as permanently provisional and, to an extent, uncertain (Ghaye & Lillyman 2000). Griffiths (1998) suggests three reasons for this. I have placed her thoughts in the context of knowledge for better team working.

- All knowledge should be open to critique from team members and others who might hold alternative views. It is therefore unwise to think that we can create a stable, unchanging knowledge base for healthcare, particularly in a rapidly changing society.
- All knowledge reflects the individual perspectives and 'positions' of the members of the team who generate it. When we try to understand and use knowledge, it is important to appreciate that perspectives and positions change.
- All knowledge is generated by people who hold certain ethical and political views. Knowledge generated by whom and for what reasons? If some kinds of team-generated knowledge are for the improvement of services and there is no consensus within the team over what constitutes improvement, or understanding of the motives of those who have generated this knowledge, then the whole situation becomes an uncertain one.

In summary, I suggest that we need to question some of our customary thinking about:

- *The sources of team knowledge.* How we come to know what we feel we need to know, whose interests these knowledges serve and their relationships with local service requirements, national and more global healthcare issues.
- *The scope of team knowledge.* What it is assumed this knowledge is able to do, how it frames and potentially resolves healthcare concerns and its relationship with local and national policy imperatives.
- *The pattern of team knowledge.* What it builds on, how it is informed from within and outside the team and the field of health. How this alters with time, and in so doing, changes or improves the relationships team members have with those they work with and care for. Finally, how it intersects with organisational changes and developments in policy from national government.

Chapter 15

Reflecting on the kinds of conversations we have with each other in a team

How might team members not only talk differently together but also talk about different things? Conversations not just about blame and deficiencies but creative ones about possibility, participation and improvement (Fredriksson & Eriksson 2003). This is an expression of doing things differently and with different people.

Difficult conversations

Sometimes over matters of patient care, about the work of colleagues, over the processes around limited resources like staffing, bed availability, breaking bad news, and so on, conversations can be difficult. They do not confine themselves to certain aspects of care and to particular people. In conversations where the issues being discussed are as important as patient care and whose outcomes are uncertain, there is the potential for staff to experience the conversation as a difficult one (Ovretveit *et al.* 1997).

A lived scenario: talk in the waiting room

On a visit to a GP surgery a receptionist declared how difficult it was for her when she had to tell people that they could not see a GP 'on demand'. This made her anxious even though she knew it was not her 'fault'. Patients were scheduled on a 10-minute booking system. She said "one patient rang me this morning, at 8.40 am wanting to see a doctor today, urgently. We've been really busy lately and it's the holiday season. The patient's regular doctor was on holiday. I could only fit her in, with another female doctor, the next day, at 10.20am". The receptionist knew she was not, in one sense, responsible for this decision. It was the first available slot. Her anxiety centred upon how the conversation made her feel about herself. She went on to explain, "I did what I could. I sensed I let the patient down. She expected something different. I'm not the kind of person who lets people down. I like to try to find a way of juggling things."

In this scenario the receptionist's self-image as a person who juggles appointments to help satisfy patient needs, conflicts with the fact that she has to say 'no, sorry not today'.

How far is talk in teams power free?

The idea of difficult conversations is illuminated further through an encounter between Sophie (a female, 30-year-old patient who suffered a serious car accident and who was in a spinal injuries unit for 3 months) and the team of professionals responsible for her care as an outpatient. Difficulty in this conversation is defined by Sophie. What follows are her reflections of a meeting with a junior doctor, a modern matron, an occupational therapist and a consultant. Some serious questions arise from the encounter.

A lived scenario: Sophie's difficult conversation

Sophie recalls:
"It was time for my first outpatient's appointment at the unit since leaving the hospital in December. Six weeks had passed and I felt that my progress had been slow but noticeable. I was steadier on my feet now but still had to use crutches for support ... and my right foot still dropped awkwardly, making me concentrate hard when I walked so that I didn't trip over. I still felt weak and could only walk for short distances at a time but I felt sure that things were moving in the right direction and that, if I persevered with my acupuncture and the physiotherapy, however painful, and kept up my own exercise regime, it would pay off.

My mood when I entered the outpatients' department was good. After a short wait I was led to the consultation room and was met by a young doctor, the matron and one of the occupational therapy team. I knew the doctor reasonably well, the matron had nursed me many times when I was a patient and the occupational therapist had taken me home when I left the hospital. We spent about 15 minutes discussing my progress and how I felt about things. We talked about life back at home, the support I was getting, my physiotherapy and the way I was coping. The conversation was positive, encouraging and supportive. Then I brought up an issue that had been worrying me for some time. It was the going back to work one. Both the doctor and sister reassured me that, although my body was slowly recovering, I needed time to get used to the traumatic changes that had taken place in the previous 5 months and to think about returning to work only when I was physically and mentally ready. The occupational therapist agreed. They did not want my progress to be hindered, particularly as my work involved sitting for long periods of time at a computer with little or no opportunities to walk, exercise and develop the wasted muscles in my legs. This was a huge relief to me and so I continued to discuss other issues.

Enter the consultant. The occupational therapist suddenly had to leave because of 'other things'. It's difficult to describe the way an atmosphere changes in a hospital when a consultant enters the room! As a patient I admire the work they do and I appreciate everything that was done for me when I was injured. BUT I still cannot come to terms with the way nothing they say is questioned or debated in front of them. Plenty is said once they disappear but never to their face. In the space of ten minutes, my sense of optimism had evaporated. Gone was the reassuring, positive, forward thinking approach. In came the conversation that was blunt, factual and unemotional. The conversation that left me distraught, angry and near to tears.

At first my progress was discussed, as before and my general well being established. Then the consultant asked,

"So are you back at work now?"
"No, not yet."
"Why not?"
"I find that I get tired very quickly at home and I'm worried that it will affect my work. I have to concentrate hard and I can't afford to make mistakes. Sitting for long periods hurts my back as well."
"What job do you do?"
"I work with computers."
"So what's the problem? You can sit. There's nothing physically stopping you from sitting at a computer is there?"
"No that's true. But it's very uncomfortable after just a short while."
"Well that's to be expected at first. You'll soon get used to it."
"But I don't feel ready to go back. I don't feel able to take on the work and all its responsibilities at the moment."
"I think you'll be fine. We'll make a note on your records that you can return to work in a week's time. Now let's have a look at that right foot, shall we?"
What else was said to me in the conversation passed in a blur. I glanced at the doctor and matron as the consultant started to talk about other matters. The doctor looked awkward. The matron sat with her eyes averted. Neither had said a word. I wanted to beg them to:
"Say something, please. Tell him that you don't think that I'm ready yet. Tell him what you told me. Tell him that the body may be recovering but it will take months for me to come to terms with the trauma. Tell him, please."
Yet I said nothing. Their faces said it all. They, in turn, were begging *me* not to say anything. How could they? He was the consultant. He had the last say. I felt the tears well-up and my throat tighten but I would not give him the pleasure . . . the pleasure of seeing me upset. Perhaps this was wrong. But this is how it was.
The consultant left the room. Both the matron and doctor looked at me for the first time.
"I'm so sorry," said the junior doctor. "I didn't expect him to make that suggestion. Thank you for not saying anything."
"I can't believe it," I said. "He just didn't want to listen to me. He is the only person I know who can make me feel so guilty and so upset. I can't imagine going back to work just yet. I don't feel ready."
The matron looked at me sympathetically and said,
"We have no choice but to write his recommendation in your notes. But what I suggest is that you go to your own doctor when you get home and explain that you do not feel strong enough to go back to work at the moment. He will then sign you off."

"Won't he have read my notes though?"

"No. But even if he has, he will make his decision based on what *you* tell him about how you feel. There's no need to discuss the conversation that you have just had with the consultant if you don't want to."

I thanked the matron and doctor for their understanding and left the hospital. Outside I broke down in tears."

What makes conversations difficult?

There are many elements to this. Sophie's conversation with staff in a multi-disciplinary team illuminates the role and power of language, the power of words that are spoken and heard. Words that are unspoken and unheard. But there is much more to learn from this scenario. What about the part played by the occupational therapist? What about what was thought and felt? The encounter reveals something about the nature and power of silence and body languages that shape and lead the conversation in different directions. In Sophie's case there were strong thoughts and emotions that she tried to conceal, feelings of guilt, vulnerability, a loss of dignity and bewilderment when the conversation she expected and hoped for, did not materialise. In the matron's and junior doctor's case there was silence, eyes conveying embarrassment and apprehension. In the consultant's view there may have been feelings of frustration or annoyance when the advice he gave was questioned. But there is much, much more in this scenario than meets the ear!

Sometimes in team talk there is a difference between what we think and what we end up saying. Also what we say is not always that which is heard. There is also a difference between what we say and what we think we have said, what we think the listener/s have heard and the actual sense they make of things. Conversations potentially become difficult when there are tensions between what a team member really thinks and what they actually say, or do not say. A team member may feel a need to share their thoughts but this is different from actually being able to do so. In difficult conversations deciding how much to say about what we are really thinking, can cause us concern and so the conversation begins to be shaped by what we feel should *not* be said. Sometimes what is said, is safe, rather than personal.

For Sophie there were at least two significant conversations going on that afternoon. The one between herself and the consultant. The other between her and other staff present. To focus on the former for a moment. There is a great deal of important work in the fields of conversational and discourse analysis and from medical sociology that provide lenses through which to try to understand what was going on between them. For example, according to Stone *et al.* (1999) there is an underlying structure to all difficult conversations. They claim that a difficult conversation is made up of three parts of what they call *conversations-within-a-conversation*.

The 'What Happened?' Conversation

Stone *et al.* (1999) suggest that most difficult conversations involve disagreement about what *has* happened, or, potentially more perplexing and value-laden, over what *should* have happened. When reflecting on 'what happened' there is usually some fuzziness over who actually said and did what. This is because the worlds we inhabit are socially constructed in particular ways, for certain reasons and purposes. The point also has something to do with memory, what we attend to and retain. 'You actually said this.' 'Oh no I didn't.' 'Oh yes you did!' Meaningful team talk should not be a pantomime, stuck over issues of who was right or wrong. For a team, there may be no disagreement over an admission or discharge process. All involved may agree that improvements can be made. The diversity of view may be over whether improving the process is worth the extra effort required and/or how best to implement this. These are not questions of right or wrong but questions of value judgement. By moving away from issues of right or wrong to those of values and judgement, we give ourselves a better chance of trying to understand how each member is making sense of the work of the team.

Assumptions are also an element of the 'what happened' part of a difficult conversation. It is unwise to assume that we know the intentions of those in our team. Intentions are often difficult to determine. Sometimes we may assume them from people's behaviour. The third and final suggestion concerns the way the attributes of blame can twist and tangle up participants in a conversation. They can add another layer of difficulty and produce disagreement, denial, defensiveness, fear, and so on. Fear of failure, of incompetence, fear of being punished, reprimanded or humiliated. In conversations infused by blame, much of the energy of staff goes into defending themselves. Being fixated by blame gets in the way of learning. A child is abused, an elderly person falls, there is an error on a drug round, and so on. We need to shift conversations so that we fix our attention on 'contribution' not on blame. In other words what happened that contributed to the incident. This is a subtle but important distinction.

The Feelings Conversation

Conversations about care can be emotional ones. Bringing up and talking about feelings can be uncomfortable. We can feel vulnerable. We can make others feel vulnerable. We can have our feelings dismissed as irrational, plain silly or listened to with real understanding. We can get feelings 'off our chest'. This might make us feel better. But what about their impact on those who are around us? Stone *et al.* (1999, p. 13) argue that '... *difficult conversations do not just involve feelings; they are at their very core about feelings. Feelings are not some noisy by-product of engaging in difficult talk, they are an integral part of the conflict. Engaging in a difficult conversation without talking about feelings is like staging an opera without the music. You'll get the plot but miss the point'.* Arguably, every difficult conversation has an affective and emotional aspect. In teams we may find ourselves thinking about how far we should express our 'true' feelings on the matters being discussed? We may think: Are my feelings valid? I wonder what others in my team are feeling?

The Identity Conversation

Here the focus of attention is upon what this conversation means to us. This may be the most subtle and challenging of all the *conversations-within-conversations* because it requires individuals and teams of health-care staff to look inward and reflect upon serious issues like 'who we are', 'how we see ourselves'. In relation to team development this is all about the team's image, professional visibility and esteem. It is also about individual members in relation with others. For example, you may think, 'I'm just seeing this conversation with my manager as asking them to reconsider what they've asked me to do, as yet another extension of my role and responsibilities'. Doing more? What if your manager doesn't see it this way? What if they see it as within your current job specification? What if your manager gives you good reasons for seeing it this way? The conversation may be about work-load, ostensibly, but what is really making you feel anxious is that your self-image and view of self-worth is on the line! This identity conversation can be a private one. A conversation we have in our heads about how far we feel good or bad about what's being said, anxious, guilty, 'balanced' about what is going on in front of us. It impacts on our sense of esteem, self-concept, efficacy, and so on.

Conversations in teams are exceedingly complex phenomena, constructed according to different conventions, ever-shifting personal intentions, consensual agreements, differences, patterns of mutual positioning with respect to rights to speak and to be heard, and obligations to listen and/or respond. The conversation this team had with Sophie is a fragmentary insight into the way healthcare professionals-with-patients create, maintain, dismantle, transform and abrogate personal and social identities and relations. We have much to learn from discursive psychology on the matter. Additionally, through the reflective lens of medical sociology we might conjecture that the consultant was making a number of 'medical moves'. One of these may well have involved *figuring*. This is a process of making people more visible as particular types of patient (Latimer 1997). Figuring patients means identifying them in particular ways and assigning them to categories such as 'good or bad', 'cheerful or moody', 'helpful or troublesome', 'self-destructive or deviant', a 'problem or awkward' patient, and so on. Unless asked we will never know how he may have been figuring Sophie, or indeed if he was. What we might say is that he had a view of her as someone ready to move forward, re-entering the world of work. Whatever sense you have made of this conversation and how this might help deepen your appreciation of the importance of a team 'talking to learn' (not learning to talk in this case), some things emerge for further reflection.

- In trying to learn from difficult conversations we should invest time in trying to understand what they mean to the participants, not in who is right and who may be wrong.
- Energy and skill might usefully be invested in trying to determine what is felt to be important to a team, not what seems to be true or false about a matter.
- Talk embodies power. We need to be aware of how this affects team working and learning.
- We need to appreciate in team talk that the talk enables and constrains action. Here attention needs to be on the influence of one on the other and vice versa. Some talk achieves closure or a level of agreement on the meaning of an event or issue, thereby enabling some kind of action to take place.
- Different disciplines have different languages. Talking in that/those language/s helps to constitute individual and team identities. These identities influence how we are perceived. This, in turn, influences how the appropriateness, legitimacy and personal significance of the person's actions are evaluated.
- In the conversation Sophie had with her team of healthcare professionals, talk was action, not inaction. When teams talk we need to bear in mind that talking can be seen as an alternative to action, to actually doing something and getting on with things. This is illustrated when teams say to me, 'Oh we haven't done anything yet, we've just been talking'. But talk can also be seen as a form of action. We would not see it this way if we did not reverse our customary linear thinking. Namely, that we move from talk to action and then to outcomes. Of course in some teams, talk and the time it takes, can be deployed 'politically'. By this I mean it is an impediment to action, soaking up precious moments that could otherwise be used to 'do something else, better, more productive'. I shall come back to this in Part Four.
- Team talk needs to have a focus on team learning. To enable this, team members need to listen to what a person is saying rather than listening to what they want to hear.

Chapter 16

Teams as a forum for asking serious questions

Burns and Grove (1993) suggest that, for the nursing profession at least, it has historically acquired knowledge through the five principle modes of tradition, authority, borrowing, trial and error, and role modelling (for a critique of these sources of knowledge see Ghaye & Lillyman 2000). Through a culture of asking questions staff make themselves more aware of the power dynamics that operate at all levels in the health service. They are able to detect the hegemonic influences that effect what they do. Hegemony is a powerful and complex word. It was the Italian political economist Antonio Gramsci (1978) who used the term to describe the process whereby ideas, structures and actions come to be seen, by the majority of people, as wholly natural, pre-specified and working in their own best interests. In fact what is really happening is that the very things that are effecting what we feel, think and do are constructed and transmitted by powerful minority interests to protect the status quo that serves their interests so well.

This is an important set of ideas and highly relevant to team working. The sinister aspect of hegemonic influences is that, over time, they become deeply embedded in the places where staff work. They become part of their cultural fabric. Part of our everyday working lives. They become the values, conventional wisdoms, customs and practices, the common-sense ways of seeing and doing things. They become part of what we take for granted. This is why asking serious questions is so important. They are a way of questioning the taken-for-grantedness of our everyday practice. The dark irony of hegemonic influences is that many healthcare workers take pride in acting on those very things that work to enslave them. A team's work ethic, commitments to each other and to patient care, often mean that they work hard to implement these customs and practices. In doing so they become willing prisoners who lock their own cell doors behind them!

Much of this work ethic is tied up with the notion of *responsibility*. For teams this is a key issue. Feeling over-responsible or under-responsible for the situations they find themselves in, usually ends up exacerbating the situation. Understanding how the 'responsibility virus' (Martin 2003) works for and against teams is critical. More of this in Part Four. At this point in the book I am simply saying that reflective teams are able to stand outside their own practice so to speak, and view it through lenses that alert them to hegemonic influences. They are able to see that certain influences can be highly corrosive and damaging to themselves and their service. A serious question therefore becomes: Whose interests are actually being served? Another is: Can we really serve the interests of 'others' if, in doing so, they harm and constrain us?

In general I would hope that the challenge implicit in a question is not being seen simply as an attack on authority or acquired wisdom but more as a way of fulfilling our:

- *moral obligation* to serve the interests of patients and clients so as to make ethical and competent decisions about how quality personalised care can be nourished and sustained;
- *personal commitment* to continue to deliver care based upon the best evidence available to us, our knowledge of what constitutes 'best practice' and that which is derived through respecting the skills, expertise and contributions of colleagues, especially when working as a member of a team; and
- *professional duty* to constantly hold under review the nature and effectiveness of our practice, a practice that needs to be lawful, safe and effective.

In being the best we can, it may be worthwhile reflecting on Salas' (1997) perceptive (and serious) question: How can you turn a team of experts into an expert team?

References

Alimo-Metcalfe, B. & Alimo-Metcalfe, J. (2003) Stamp of greatness. *Health Service Journal*, 26 June, 28–32.

Amason, A.C., Thompson, K.R., Hochwarter, W.A. & Harrison, A.W. (1995) Conflict: an important dimension in successful management teams. *Organizational Dynamics*, **24**(2), 20–35.

Audit Commission (2002) *Recruitment and Retention: A Public Service Workforce for the 21st Century*. Audit Commission, London.

Barbour, A. (1995) *Caring for Patients: A Critique of the Medical Model*. Stanford University Press, Stanford.

Barnes, B. (2000) *Understanding Agency: Social Theory and Responsible Action*. Sage, London.

Beresford, P. (2000) Service users' knowledge's and social work theory: conflict or collaboration? *British Journal of Social Work* **30**, 489–503.

Betts, C. (2003) Hutt pushes partnership but closes door on foundations. *Health Service Journal*, 15 May.

Bleakley, A. (2000) Writing with invisible ink: narrative, confessionalism and reflective practice. *Reflective Practice* **1**(1), 11–24.

Boaden N, & Leaviss, J. (2000) Putting teamwork in context. *Medical Education* **34**(11), 921–927.

Brower, M.J. (1995) Empowering teams: what, why and how. *Empowerment in Organizations* **3**(1), 13–25.

Burns, N. & Grove, S. (1993) *The Practice of Nursing Research: Conduct, Critique and Utilization*. Harcourt Brace, London.

Calman, K. & Hine, D. (1995) *A Policy Framework for Commissioning Cancer Services. A Report by the Expert Advisory Group for the DoH*. Department of Health, London.

Carr, D. (1992) Practical enquiry, values and the problem of educational theory. *Oxford Review of Education* **18**(3), 241–51.

Castka, P., Bamber, C.J. & Sharp, J. M. (2003) Measuring teamwork culture: the use of a modified EFQM model. *Journal of Management Development* **22**(2), 149–170.

Chambers, R. (1998) *Challenging the Professions*. Intermediate Technology, London.

Collins, J. (2001) *Good to Great: Why Some Companies Make the Leap ... and Others Don't*. HarperBusiness, New York.

Collison, C. & Parcell, G. (2001) *Learning to Fly: Practical Lessons from One of the World's Leading Knowledge Companies*. Capstone, Oxford.

Commission for Health Improvement (2003) *A Report on the NHS: Getting Better?* CHI, London.

Cooke, B. & Kothari, U. (eds) (2001) *Participation: The New Tyranny?* Zed Books, London.

Dawson, S. & Smith, T. (2002) *Evaluating the Impact of the NHS Clinical Support Team's Clinical Governance Programme*. University of Cambridge, Judge Institute of Management, Cambridge

Department of Health (1997) *The New NHS: Modern and Dependable*. DoH, London.

Department of Health (1998) *A First Class Service: Quality in the NHS*. DoH, London.

Department of Health (1999) *Making a Difference: Strengthening the Nursing, Midwifery and Health Visiting Contribution to Health and Healthcare*. DoH, London.

Department of Health (2000) *Working Together: Staff Involvement, A Self Assessment Tool*. DoH, Leeds.

Department of Health (2001a) *Working Together – Learning Together: A Framework for Lifelong Learning in the NHS*. DoH, London.

Department of Health (2001b) *Working Lives Programmes for Change Positively Diverse*. DoH, London.

Department of Health (2002a) *Liberating the Talents: Helping Primary Care Trusts and Nurses to Deliver the NHS Plan*. DoH, London.

Department of Health (2002b) *Managing for Excellence in the NHS*. DoH, London.

Department of Health (2002c) *Shifting the Balance of Power: The Next Steps*. DoH, London.

Department of Health. (2002d) *Improving Working Lives for the Allied Health Professions and Healthcare Scientists*. DoH, London.

Department of Health (2003) *Raising Standards. Improving Performance in the NHS*. DoH, London.

Dombeck, M. (1997) Professional personhood: training, territoriality and tolerance. *Journal of Interprofessional Care* **11**, 9–21.

Duckworth, L. & Morris, N. (2001) Conspiracy of silence behind the needless deaths of 35 infants. *The Independent*, 19 July.

Eggensperger, J.D. (2004) How far is too far? Lessons for business from ultra-high-performing military teams. *Team Performance Management*, **10**(3/4), 53–59.

Elston, S. & Holloway, I. (2001) The impact of recent primary care reforms in the UK on interprofessional working in primary care centres. *Journal of Interprofessional Care* **15**(1), 19–27.

Fleming, J.L. & Monda-Amaya, L.E. (2001) Process variables critical for team effectiveness: a Delphi study of wraparound team members. *Remedial and Special Education* **22**(3), 158–171.

Flory, M. (1998) International team effectiveness. *Journal of Managerial Psychology* **13**(3/4), 225–229.

Freeman, M. & Procter-Childs, T. (1998) Visions of teamwork: the realities of an interdisciplinary approach. *British Journal of Therapy and Rehabilitation* **5**, 616–618.

Freeman, M., Miller, C. & Ross, N. (2000) The impact of individual philosophies of teamwork on multi-professional practice and the implications for education. *Journal of Interprofessional Care* **14**(3), 237–247.

Freeth, D. (2001) Sustaining interprofessional collaboration. *Journal of Interprofessional Care* **15**(1), 38–46.

Fredriksson, L. & Eriksson, K. (2003) The ethics of the caring conversation. *Nursing Ethics: An International Journal for Health Care Professionals* **10**(2), 138–148.

Ghaye, T (forthcoming) *Building the Reflective Healthcare Organisation*. Blackwell Publishing, Oxford.

Ghaye, T. (2005) Editorial: reflection for spiritual practice? *Reflective Practice* **5**(3), 291–295.

Ghaye, T. & Lillyman, S. (2000) *Reflection: Principles and Practice for Healthcare Professionals*. Quay Books, Wiltshire.

Ghaye, T. & Lillyman, S. (2001) *Learning Journals and Critical Incidents: Reflective Practice for Health Care Professionals*. Quay Books, Wiltshire.

Gilbert, J.H.V., Camp II, R.D., Cole, C.D., Bruce, C., Fielding, D.W. & Stanton, S.J. (2000) Preparing students for interprofessional team work in health care. *Journal of Interprofessional Care* **14**(3), 223–235.

Gladwell, M. (2000) *The Tipping Point*. Little Brown, Boston.

Gladwell, M. (2002) The personnel department. *The New Yorker*, 22 July, 28–30.

Goldhammer, R. (1966) *A critical analysis of supervision of instruction in the Harvard-Lexington Summer Programme*. Unpublished PhD thesis, Harvard University, Boston.

Gramsci, A. (1978) *Selections from the Prison Notebooks*. Lawrence & Wishart, London.

Griffiths, M. (1998) *Educational Research for Social Justice: Getting off the Fence*. Open University Press, Buckingham.

Greco, M. & Carter, M. (2002) *Improving Practice Questionnaire (IPQ) Tool Kit*. Aeneas Press, Bodmin.

Handy, C. (1996) *Beyond Certainty*. Arrow Business Books, London.

Hardie, R. (2000) A caring moment with Peter. In *Caring Moments: The Discourse of Reflective Practice*. (eds T. Ghaye & S. Lillyman). Quay Books, Wiltshire.

Harré, R. & Langenhove, L. (1999) *Positioning Theory*. Blackwell, Oxford.

Hickey, S. & Mohan, G. (eds) (2004) *Participation: From Tyranny to Transformation?* Zed Books, London.

Higgs, J. & Titchen, A. (2001) *Professional Practice in Health, Education and the Creative Arts*. Blackwell Science, Oxford.

Hitchcock, D. & Willard, M. (1995). *Why Teams Fail and What to Do About it*. Irwin, Chicago.

Hunt, C. & Sampson, F. (1998) *The Self on the Page*. Jessica Kingsley, London.

Imai, M. (1986) *Kaizen, the Key to Japan's Competitive Success*, McGraw-Hill, New York.

Institute of Health Management (2002) Teamwork is vital. *Health Management*, November, 7.

IRP-UK (2005) *TA²LK: The Essence of Improvement*. The Institute of Reflective Practice, IRP-UK, Gloucester.

Jackson, C.J. (2002) Predicting team performance from a learning process model. *Journal of Managerial Psychology* **17**(1), 6–13.

James, K. (1999) Issues in management research, and the value of psychoanalytic perspective: a case study in organisational stress in a Japanese company. Presented at the Conference of the International Society for the Psychoanalytic Study of Organisations, Toronto, 25–27 June.

Johns, C. (2002) *Guided Reflection: Advancing Practice*. Blackwell, Oxford.

Jones, B. & Jones, G. (1996) *Earth Dance Drum: A Celebration of Life*. Commune-A-Key, Salt Lake City.

Katzenbach, J.R. & Smith, D.K. (2003) *The Wisdom of Teams*. Harper Business Essentials, London.

Kember, D., Jones, A., Loke, A.Y., McKay, J., Sinclair, K., Tse, H., Webb, C., Wong, F.K.Y. & Yeung, E. (2001) *Reflective Teaching and Learning in the Health Professions*. Blackwell Science, Oxford.

Kipp, M.F. & Kipp, M.A. (2000) Of teams and teambuilding. *Team Performance Management* **6**(7/8), 138–139.

Laidler, P. (1991) Adults and how to become one. *Therapy Weekly* **17**(35), 4.

Kotter, J. & Cohen, D. (2002) *The Heart of Change*. Harvard Business School Press, Boston.

Kübler Ross, E. (1969) *On Death and Dying*. Macmillan, London.

Lamont, G. (2002) *The Spirited Organisation: Success Stories of Soul-Friendly Companies*. Hodder and Stoughton, London.

Langer, A. (2005) *IT and Organizational Learning: Managing Change through Technology and Education*. Routledge, Oxford.

Latimer, J. (1997) Giving patients a future: the constituting of classes in an acute medical unit. *Sociology of Health and Illness* **19**(2), 160–185.

Lowe, F. & O'Hara, S. (2000). Multi-disciplinary team working in practice: managing the transition. *Journal of Interprofessional Care* **14**(3), 270–279.

Lundin, W & Lundin, K. (1996) How to grow dream teams. *R & D Innovator* **5**(2), 119.

Mallik, M., Hall, C. & Howard, D. (eds) (1998) *Nursing Knowledge and Practice: A Decision-Making Approach*. Bailliere Tindall, London.

Martin, R. (2003) *The Responsibility Virus*. Prentice Hall, Harlow.

Maslow, A.H. (1987) *Motivation and Personality*, 3rd edn. Harper & Row, New York.

Mayeroff, M. (1971) *On Caring*. Harper and Row, New York.

McIntyre, I. (2003) Do the knowledge. *Health Management* May, 10–11.

McNiff, J. & Whitehead, J. (2001) *Action Research in Organisations*. Routledge, London.

McNiff, J. & Whitehead, J. (2002) *Action Research: Principles and Practice*, 2nd edn. Taylor and Francis, Oxford.

Molyneux, J. (2001) Interprofessional teamworking: what makes them work well? *Journal of Interprofessional Care* **15**(91), 29–35.

NHS Modernisation Agency (2003) *Improving Performance in the NHS*. Department of Health, London.

Noddings, N. (1986) *Caring: A Feminine Approach to Ethic and Moral Education*. University of California Press, Berkeley.

Nonaka, I. & Takeuchi, H. (1995) *The Knowledge-Creating Company. How Japanese Companies Create the Dynamics of Innovation*. Oxford University Press, Oxford.

Novak, J. (1998) *Learning, Creating and Using Knowledge*. Lawrence Erlbaum, London.

NMC (2002) *Supporting Nurses and Midwives through Lifelong Learning*. Nursing and Midwifery Council, London.

Offenbeek, M. (2001) Processes and outcomes of team learning. *European Journal of Work and Organisational Psychology* **10**(3), 303–317.

Oliver, S. & Tonks, P. (1998) Team briefing – helping to rediscover the road to Utopia. *Health Manpower Management* **24**(2), 69–75.

Ovretveit, J., Mathias, P. & Thompson, T. (1997) *Interprofessional Working for Health and Social Care*. Macmillan, London.

Parkinson, F. (1997) *Critical Incident Debriefing: Understanding and Dealing with Trauma*. Souvenir Press, London.

Peters, T. & Waterman, R. (1982) *In Search of Excellence: Lessons from America's Best-run Companies*. Harper and Row, New York.

Phillips, J. (2000) *Contested Knowledge: A Guide to Critical Theory*. Zed Books, London.

Polanyi, M. (1958) *Personal Knowledge*. Oxford University Press, Oxford.

Polley, D. & Ribbens, B. (1998) Sustaining self-managed teams: a process approach to team wellness. *Team Performance Management* **4**(1), 3–21.

Pook, L. (2004) How can we work as a team? *Professional Nurse* **20**(2), 56.

Prasad, B. (2001) What management style is considered best for a team-based organisation and why? *International Journal of Value-Based Management* **14**, 59–77.

Rabey, G. (2001) Is the team building industry nearing the apex of its S curve? *Team Performance Management: An International Journal* **7**(7/8), 112–116.

Rayner, S.R. (1996) *Team Traps: Survival Stories and Lessons for Team Disasters, Near-Misses, Mishaps, and Other Near-Death Experiences*. John Wiley & Sons, New York.

Rickards, T. & Moger, S. (1999) *Handbook for Creative Team Leaders*. Gower, Aldershot.

Robbins, H. & Finley, M. (1995) *Why Teams Fail: What Went Wrong and How to Make it Right*. Peterson's/Pacesetter Books, Princeton, New Jersey.

Rolfe, G. & Fulbrook, P. (eds) (1998) *Advanced Nursing Practice*. Butterworth-Heinemann, Oxford.

Royal College of Nursing (2003) *The Future Nurse*. www.rcn.org.uk/downloads/congress(2003)/ future-nurse.pdf

Royal College of Nursing. *Leadership Project and LEO Programme*. www.nursingleadership.co.uk/ren_leo.htm

Runnymede Bulletin (1997) A new vision for Britain. *Runnymede Bulletin*, 306.

Rushmer, R. (1997) What happens to the team during teambuilding? Examining the change process that helps to build a team. *Journal of Management Development* **16**(5), 316–327.

Salas, E. (1997) How can you turn a team of experts into an expert team? In *Naturalistic Decision Making* (eds C.E. Zsambok & G. Klein). Lawrence Erlbaum, Mahwah.

Scholtes, O., Joiner, B. & Streibel, B. (1996), *The Team Handbook*. Oriel.

Schön, D. (1983) *The Reflective Practitioner*. Basic Books, New York.

Schön, D. (ed.) (1991) *The Reflective Turn: Case Studies in and on Educational Practice*. Teachers College Press, New York.

SCOPME (1997) *Multiprofessional Working and Learning: Sharing the Educational Challenge*. Consultation Paper. The Standing Committee on Postgraduate Medical and Dental Education, London.

Scott, C. (2003) It's time to invest in our nursing teams. Editorial. *Professional Nurse* **18**(12), 662.

Sheard, A. G. & Kakabadse, A. P. (2002) From loose groups to effective teams: the nine key factors of the team landscape. *Journal of Management Development* **21**(2), 133–151.

Stone, D. Patton, B. & Heen, S. (1999). *Difficult Conversations: How to Discuss What Matters Most*. Michael Joseph, London.

Stott, K. & Walker, A. (1995) *Teams, Teamwork and Teambuilding*. Prentice-Hall, London.

Street, A. (1995) *Nursing Replay: Researching Nursing Culture Together*. Churchill Livingstone, London.

Stronach, I. & MacLure, M. (1997) *Educational Research Undone: The Postmodern Embrace*. Open University Press, Buckingham.

Taylor, J. (2002) 'It's all I ever wanted to do'. *Nursing Times* **98**(50), 42–43.

Telleria, K.M., Little, D. & MacBryde, J. (2002) Managing processes through teamwork. *Business Process Management Journal* **8**(4), 338–350.

Tuckman, B.W. (1965) Development sequences in small groups. *Psychology Bulletin* **63**(6), 384–399.

von Krogh, G., Ichijo, K. & Nonaka, I. (2000) *Enabling Knowledge Creation: How to Unlock the Mystery of Tacit Knowledge and Release the Power of Innovation*. Oxford University Press, Oxford.

Wakhlu, A. (1999) *Managing from the Heart: Unfolding Spirit in People and Organisations.* Response Books, New Delhi.

Wenger, E. (2002) *Communities of Practice: Learning, Meaning and Identity.* Cambridge University Press, Cambridge.

Wenger, E., McDermott, R. & Snyder, W.M. (2002) *A Guide to Managing Knowledge: Cultivating Communities of Practice.* Harvard Business School Press, Boston.

Whitehead, J. (1993) *The Growth Of Educational Knowledge: Creating Your Own Living Educational Theories.* Hyde, Bournemouth.

Whitehead, J. (2000) How do I improve my practice? Creating and legitimating an epistemology of practice. *Reflective Practice* **1**(1), 91–104.

Whitehead, J. with Johns, C. (2000) A response to Whitehead, and a reply. *Reflective Practice* **1**(1), 105–112.

Part Four
About DEVELOPING REFLECTIVE TEAMS

Chapter 17
How to get there

Part Two of this book was *about reflection*. It explored some of the interests and practices of it. Part Three was *about teams* and ways of being the best we can. These two parts inform this final section of the book. Here the central question, 'How can we develop reflective health-care teams that are able to sustain high quality, personalised care?' is addressed through a form of *disciplined action* (see Part Three) called **TA²LK** (IRP-UK 2005). It has been developed with staff and service users in healthcare since 1995. It has five mutually supporting elements which encourage:

- *learning through* the interests and practices of reflection;
- *learning through* working together, in teams;
- *learning through* a facilitated process based upon the idea of team wellness and the healthy team.

TA²LK is a fully validated, evidence-based, facilitated team learning process. It enables 'serious questions' about the quality of healthcare services to be asked, and creative responses to them imagined, talked about, planned for and evaluated. Of course, turning better thinking into improved services is a difficult thing. But those engaged with **TA²LK** accept the responsibilities of team-organised learning and responsible action. They work out how they might engineer and sustain 'creative spaces' for each other so that they can determine, manage and regulate what they wish to improve and sustain in their work. **TA²LK** is about healthcare teams engaging in *conversations of possibility*. It is the possibility of improving practice. Part Four draws upon the work of staff at the international Institute of Reflective Practice-UK, its healthcare partners and affiliated consultants during the period 1999–2004. The data base constitutes work with 753 teams in health and social care in the United Kingdom and 3211 service users.

The development of **TA²LK** has been influenced by a number of significant research literatures, and staff and service user experiences. For example, with regard to published work, it has been influenced by Harré's 'personal being' and the position he adopts, namely that 'the primary human reality is persons in conversation' (Harré, 1983, p. 58), and by Freire (1972), who believed that through dialogue people are supposed to create new understandings that are explicitly critical and aimed at action. In the context of developing reflective teams, this means that staff reject the role of 'puppet' and 'object' and become much more proactive, trying to shape their own destiny. It has also been influenced by Gadamer (1979, p. 347), who describes conversation in this way. '*It is a process of two people understanding each other. Thus it is a characteristic of every true conversation that each opens himself to the other person, truly accepts his point of view as worthy of consideration and gets inside the other to such an extent that he understands not a particular individual, but what he says.*'

The point Gadamer (1979) is making, that is so central to the **TA²LK** process, is that knowledge for 'better practice' is not a fixed thing or a commodity, 'out there' waiting to be discovered. It arises out of inter-action within and between teams. Gadamer used the very helpful notion of 'horizons of understanding' in explaining his case. For example, that through conversation the aim is not to 'win the argument' (always) but to advance understanding. Our personal horizon of understanding is the range of vision we have when in conversation with another. It is what we can see and understand (given our prejudices, biases, values, expect-ations, pre-judgements, and so on) from a particular vantage point or at a particular time. Gadamer argues that when in conversation we need to try to understand a horizon that is not our own, in relation to our own. This is not a process of win-lose, agree/disagree, but a process of dis-covering and advancing our understanding of other people's standpoint and horizon. Burbules (1993), who talks about a conversation being a particular kind of social relationship that entails certain virtues and emotions, also had an influence on TA²LK. Referring to 'hope', Burbules stresses that we need to engage in conversations *in the hope* that they hold a possibility that we will learn or gain something from them.

These conceptions of talking and conversing may be in the realm of the 'ideal' for some teams. Conversations based upon mutual respect, a willingness to listen, to risk airing ones honest opinions, to appreciate and learn from diversity, may not be commonplace where you work. This ideal was described by Habermas (1984) as an 'ideal speech situation'. It is where those involved in a conversation have an equality of chances to take part in a meaningful exchange and where the conversation is un-constrained and not distorted. This idea of an 'ideal speech situation' provides us with a way of identifying and understanding the distortions that actually exist in the everyday work of teams. For example, distor-tions due to patterns of power associated with learned behaviours, defensiveness, and so on. Distortions of the ideal speech situation can be brought about by the language/s we use. Sometimes language is used to 'keep staff at bay', out there, to deliberately mystify. On other occa-sions the use of more inclusive language unifies, engages and opens-up rather than closing out the constructive exploration of ideas and issues.

Research from the following peer-reviewed journals also informed the development of **TA²LK.**

- *The European Journal of Work and Organisational Psychology*
- *The Journal of Management Inquiry*

- *Group and Organisation Management*
- *Journal of Management Development*
- *Empowerment in Organisations*
- *Strategic Change*
- *Journal of Organisational Behaviour*
- *Journal of Workplace Learning*
- *Journal of Managerial Psychology*
- *Journal of Organisational Change Management*
- *The Learning Organisation*
- *Participation and Empowerment: An International Journal*

Finally, work from the United Nations Research Institute for Social Development (UNRISD) and the United Nations Educational, Scientific and Cultural Organisation (UNESCO) 'Culture and Development programme 1997–2003' was consulted.

Chapter 18

TA²LK and reflective conversations of possibility

The distilled essence of these literatures helped formulate a **TA²LK** process requiring habits of mind, a code of situated ethics, intellectual dispositions and team practices that enable the effective participation, of members and service users, in *conversations of possibility*. Much of this is not 'there in advance' but has to be created and learned as staff go along. In terms of *disciplined actions* these conversations require:

- Respectful understanding of where participants are 'coming from'. This is about understanding the backgrounds and diverse views held by members of teams and their service users. In significant ways these affect the commitments members make to team working and learning and the choices they exercise in specific contexts.
- An acceptance of some responsibility for trying to make these conversations 'fair'. Fairness demands opportunity. Sometimes we slide into talking about 'them', often because we feel this is easier than talking about us and me. Often the 'them' are those colleagues and users who have neither the skills nor the confidence to enter into such a conversation or enter a public forum, even as a listener.
- An understanding of the subtleties of language (Daly 1993). **TA²LK** provides opportunities for staff to engage in at least five kinds of language. (i) A *scientific language* about the validity of the improvement data gathered, how systematically it has been done and its potential generalisability. (ii) A *constructivist language*, where participant subjectivities are acknowledged and valued. (iii) An *artistic language* that enables staff to be creative and discuss new possibilities for better practice. (iv) A *critical change language* to do with persuasion, influence and overcoming resistance. (v) A *pragmatic and utilitarian language* about the way better team learning makes a difference to services.
- Listening with care but also listening for understanding, not for confirmation that we are 'always right'. These actions also include an appreciation that diversity within a team is not synonymous with discord and disharmony. Arguably, being positive about diversity is a critical attribute of a 'modern' NHS team.
- Self-expression and thinking before we talk, not being over-talkative, taking turns and exercising our moral right to explain what we think and feel in the company of those who value what it is we have to say.
- Interaction with other participants where there is a shared responsibility for getting something out of the conversation, resisting the

temptation to stereotype staff and service users and being aware of who is and is not taking a part in the conversation.

- Reflection on how far participants engage in reflective conversations as learners, not just as knowers.

Appreciating some qualities of a reflective team

What follows is a conversation between myself, some members of a district nursing team and one of their patients. The team work in a densely populated urban area. The conversation enables us to appreciate many of the key issues and qualities (which are in italics) about the nature of reflective healthcare teams? The nursing team were engaging with the **TA²LK** process.

Conversations with Doris, Dot and a district nursing team

Doris had been a team leader for 15 years. Seventy-five per cent of her work was clinical. There were 11 staff in the team, six trained nurses and five auxiliary nurses, with a mix of full- and part-time staff. There is Doris, an 'F grade', four 'E grades (one called 'Davinia' or Little Whirlwind) and five others.

> **Tony:** *Tell me a little bit about your team Doris. Paint a picture of them in words please.*
>
> **Doris:** Well they're a very together team and very loyal to one another and to myself, but also very able and *capable of challenging each other's practice and myself.* I think some outsiders call it a scary team. I think that's partly because, through reflection and lots of talking and listening, we are now actually able to, sort of, not just challenge ourselves, but other people. We used to go to our GP practice meetings, and the GP that leads would always have something to moan about, and it starts with the district nurses, basically, and it used to be that we'd sit there and they'd say to me "Doris, you've got to tell them this and you've got to tell them that." But I can't get a word in edgeways now because they say it themselves. I guess they feel stronger. They're happier with their practice. I feel that *they've been empowered really.* They are a stronger team but maybe they come across as being angry too. Some people don't like being challenged so that could be why they get interpreted that way. Some people say it's a scary team and I guess there are some characters, that could be scary, but it depends what they're talking about. If we're talking about patient care they're *very passionate, want to do their best and want what is best and what is right for the patients.* That's the main purpose. That's what we're here for. We feel it's important that patients know what we're here for ... for them. I don't tell them what to do ... *we share and discuss everything.* Another team leader said to me that I was giving them enough rope and that they would hang me. I challenged that. I know me and I know all the team, they wouldn't hang me, *they're very trusting sort of people and open and honest.*

Tony: You mentioned the word trust there. How have you come to trust each other in the ways you do?

Doris: We work together. I always stress this. And if somebody's not sure about something *we can always call upon another team member for help and support* and that goes for me too. I don't know everything, none of us do, so we will call upon others for advice. We feel that the ultimate object about being here, is the patient, that's the main thing for us and if something isn't working out for somebody, then we need to challenge that. We have grown in our confidence and feel, almost empowered really to do that challenging in the confines of our little office, that we've now got for our *reflective sessions*. We now have the safety to do that. We can say things that will remain in that room and are left behind at night. I try to encourage people to *say what's on their mind, ask questions* while they are thinking about them. I guess it's partly working together but also *knowing each other's style, temperament and ways of working*. I encourage everyone to get to know each other's capabilities and some people are more capable of some things than others and vice versa. *We feel safe to say 'I can't do that'*. To admit that we can't do something or know something. There are some things I don't like doing because I don't feel I pass on to patients the confidence in what I do. I will do it and the patients don't always know, at least I hope they don't.

Tony: You described your team as an empowered one. If I were a member of your team, how would I know I was in an empowered team as opposed to being in some other kind of team I wonder?

Doris: I think it's about expectations. They have *high expectations of myself as a team leader and of each other*. If they want something and they can't get it, or they have to go through somebody to get it because that's better for a patient, they'll sit down and say "How are we going to get this for that patient?" *We learn from each other's ideas and then share things around*. We've had problems with a very large lady (Dot) who needs a bed and it's not really for any medical condition, but because she's overweight. It's now getting difficult. She will become a nursing problem, so we sat down and discussed as a team how we could best put this to the equipment stores management and somebody said, "I'll set the letter out because I'm better at that". Two said, "We know the lady really well so we'll talk about what she really needs" and I read the letter. So it was a joint thing. There was never any question that we wouldn't be able to get that for the patient. We just go for it. If it had not been taken on board by the equipment store it would have been taken further. *This positive attitude is part of the psyche of the team now*. They don't even think that they wouldn't be able to achieve something. There's nothing that isn't within our grasp if it is for patient care. Years gone by we'd have put up with things. Thought that's not possible. But unless we push the boundaries then it's not going to happen. If we shout about patients first then it's difficult for people to argue. *Our reflective sessions have helped us find our voice. We've got to know the political language though and we're more persuasive now. We've learnt this together.*

Tony: You are describing your team as an empowered one and your job title is that of 'team leader'. So I wonder what leaders of empowered teams actually have to do?

Doris: I think it's *just being* there sometimes, with them *physically and emotionally* and *trying things out together*. Sometimes they can run off the rails a bit and I gently remind them that they have the capabilities and *letting them know that they're doing a good job*. Giving them the freedom to get on with their work, not always watching over them. Not controlling them. Encouraging them to organise themselves. Sometimes this is a bit scary, but *we always reflect on things together*, so we are always thinking about what steps we've taken and what steps to take in the future. *Reflection helps us to find our way forward.* They function really well like this and I sometimes think that they don't really need me. But I'll go on holiday and come back and they'll say, "I'm so glad to see you", and they tell me everything they've done. They like to tell me and I say you've done great holding everything together. They don't need me but they don't realise that, which is quite nice. Some say they need me for *reassurance*. I guess, dealing with the 'organisation', communications with senior management and directing things from time to time. *I'm quite placid and quiet as team leaders go* I guess and they are a strong lot. Sometimes they will shout so loud they can't be heard and I tone it down so people will listen far better. It's only because they're passionate. Sometimes I watch people who are a bit fiery and wish I could have a bit of that. But I don't think you need to be a larger than life kind of character as a leader. You don't have to match the fiery-ness of team members. All you'd get is a bigger fire!

Tony: How far do you think the team need you to give them emotional support?

Doris: I think so at times, inevitably. I guess we all sort of *feel like a family*. It's that safety net. We've had some real sad stories, personal happenings on the team. People have been ill and deaths and I was generally the first to know, even before their families sometimes. That isn't being a team leader, that's *being a friend, caring for each other*, within the team as well. I think the emotional need is nice. It's nice to be close to people. But we talk about the need to have the ability to stand back ... and closeness wouldn't come in the way. I could go and baby-sit for one of them, and they'll say, "I really disagree with what you're doing Doris" and that is absolutely fine. I welcome that. I would hate to think that just because I'm a friend they wouldn't be able to challenge me. That just because I'm a team leader I couldn't be questioned. *We care for each other but we also confront each other as well, but in a positive way.*

Tony: Everything you've said, up till now, has been your perception of the team. Can I turn it around a bit and look at things from a patient perspective? How do you think the patient you talked about earlier (Dot) might describe you and your team?

Doris: She's one of those patients that has a little name for some people. She will describe people on the team and I know who they are by their names. 'Little whirlwind', who is full of energy and rushes around. She knows her name is 'Little Whirlwind' in that house and I think it's probably helped her in a way. She said "I know I do it. I charge in and out." She knows it's all down to her star sign. It's part of her make up. Dot's a bit of a controller, but worth listening to.

Tony: How do you think she might describe you?

Doris: I've asked her that. She said, "What could I say about you". To my face she would only say nice things. I think she would say that I was quite quiet, and not at all like her! When she herself was in management she was obviously not quiet at all. She will say to me, "Why haven't you shouted at them about this and that", and "Why don't you tell them?" ... and "If you just did it yourself then it would get done quicker". She knows that I'm the team leader and she knows they know I'm the leader. She knows I don't wear it on my sleeve. I'm very different to her in my views I think. I don't know what else she would say. I'd be interested to know.

So I arranged to make a visit to Dot. She lived in a semi-detached council-owned house with her husband Stan and a small, friendly dog called Buster. Each room was a treasure trove of memorabilia of days gone by, of holidays together, family occasions and objects, large and small, which collectively signified the rich and colourful life Dot and Stan were living. After many cups of tea and attention shared between Buster and Stan's running commentary on the cricket test match, Dot and I engaged in a conversation, which lasted all afternoon. Parts of it are presented here.

Tony: What do you feel about Doris's team?
Dot: Doris's team are marvellous, you can't fault them. I've been with her team longer than anybody and they've been marvellous to me. I've been really ill and I've been rushed to hospital and brought back and they've been very good to Stan who's a very sick man, because he suffers with schizophrenia. He wouldn't harm you or me but he's a manic depressant. You've got to reassure him all of the time. He's got a bowel problem, a heart problem, angina, and diabetes... and he's got typhoids! Doris looks after him marvellously. I don't know if it's Doris's training or her personality. You get some staff and they say, "Roll over Dot" and they don't give me time. I suffer with gout and arthritis and sometimes my limbs are painful and they don't realise how tender I am. They may be short of time or they just want to get finished, but they push me and I'm not always ready for that. I don't get that with Doris's team at all. If they think I can't manage they'll help me.

Tony: When do you see staff in Doris's team?
Dot: They usually come about 10.30. If they come at 10.15 I say "Did you come in the middle of the night?" Or if they come late I'd say "Good heavens I'm ready for my supper!" I call Davinia, 'Little Whirlwind'

Tony: Oh, so you've names for people?
Dot: Some of them yes, Little Whirlwind's got too much to say and rushes around. She just rushes around causing a draft. Sue's a good nurse, bright and happy ... I call her Sunshine. Josie is a clever one. She can turn things around and see things from other people's point of view. Her name is Wise Owl. Sarah is also a very good little nurse although she's very young ... I call her Little Lamb. Then there's Fee, who I call a Racehorse because she comes in and it's all go, go, go! And of course Little Whirlwind. I tell them off if I think they're not right.

Tony: How do you think staff in Doris's team see her?
Dot: She's *very respected*, but not tough enough. *Quiet.* Too quiet at times I think. I think she's very loved and they're a happy team. She cares for people but sometimes other people do the ruling part. It's all Little Whirlwind's fault. I told her if she wants the boss's job to go and take her exams ... I think Doris is a lady. People who are a bit sterner can try and undermine her authority. It wouldn't be any of the others, just Little Whirlwind. Do you know Little Whirlwind? Sometimes I call Little Whirlwind, 'The Shadow' as well, because she's always in Doris's shadow.

Tony: How far do you see Doris as a leader?
Dot: To a point. She's not tough enough though. You've got to be tough haven't you?

Tony: Do you need to be tough to be a leader?

Dot: Yes of course. That's what it means. Yes … it is. But if things go on she will tackle it in her way. She won't make a song and dance about it. And she doesn't let things get out of hand. If something crops up she tackles it and doesn't leave it until it gets bigger and harder. Well she's probably much better at it than me. They put me in charge in 1956/57. I was still quite young then. We were allowed 15 minutes break, but the superintendent boss said one day, "If you all work hard you can have 20 minutes." After 20 minutes nobody moved, so I went to my desk and banged a ruler on it "You should all be ashamed of yourselves," I said, "If you're not going to go back to work on time, then we'll work by the rules in the future and have only 15 minutes." They immediately got back to work. They didn't talk to me for a while … but that's how it was.

After my conversation with Dot, I arranged to meet with Davinia, one of the district nursing team and the one Dot referred to as 'Little Whirlwind'. We chatted about a range of things, including how she saw her role within the team, her sense of identity, self-worth and her work with her patients. The conversation lasted for 90 minutes. Parts of it are presented here.

Tony: How do you see Doris as a team leader?

Davinia: She's got lots of qualities that I admire but sometimes I get frustrated with her because she's too calm! I want her to get annoyed with people sometimes because I think they're not pulling their weight or taking too long to get on with things. I would tell them straight and not spend time trying to understand everyone's point of view like Doris does. Sometimes you just need to be blunt with people, don't you?

Another thing. *She would never ask any of us to do something she wouldn't be prepared to have a go at herself.* She's a lot more open than me. She's *happy to be open and say what she feels* she can do and what she feels we can do together. That takes a bit of courage I guess.

We're *different people really and we know it. But this doesn't mean it gets in the way.* I'm a bit loud I know at times. I have been known to get very passionate about what we do. But Doris just let's me say my piece, and we go from there. She's sensitive that way. She's different from others I've worked with. Special. *She reads things well, reads situations well* … and only *really speaks sometimes, when she has something to say.* She doesn't just mouth-off like … well I do this sometimes I know. *She reads our mood well.* She's a reader and a good team leader

Tony: How would you describe the way you are in the team?

Davinia: Ummmm … well I think I'm different from some of the others. *I'm very keen to do the best I can for my patients*, as we all are … and I guess I have lots of energy … well that's how I think others see me. I'm not afraid to say what I think … its' important this … Doris is always saying that we should speak our minds. This way we get to know what we are all thinking and we have some good team meetings. So *no one is really afraid to say their piece … and we get a lot of good ideas this way* … you know about what we can do for our patients … how we can do things better … whether it's about our big continence case load … that's a hot topic for us right now … or anything really.

Tony: Would you say the team is made up of a lot of personalities?

Davinia: Oh yes … *we're all different in our ways, but we are all the same over some things* if you know what I mean. We all reflect on our work … we have learned to do this more, over the last couple of years. We always did it but now it's much better ... we do it differently in our team meetings. We are more focused and we support each other even if we don't agree with everyone. We aren't afraid of suggesting things. We share things around and no one gets too precious ... if one of the girls can't manage to do something, then we all try to help. I guess others would say I'm quite loud. I love my work and this team but I am a bit impatient ... yes ... I think ... only because I want the best. When we make a decision about something then, I say, it's into action ... and let's get on with it. We talk a lot and we get on with things.

There is much to learn from these conversations. We can discern some of the qualities of a reflective team. We can spot them in relation to comments that fall into three broad clusters. Comments about:

- patterns of relationships ('W*e share and discuss everything*');
- difference ('W*e are different but the same*'); and
- doing their best for their patients ('W*e want what is best and what is right for our patients*').

In the **TA²LK** process, comments in the first cluster form part of team learning within their 'care zone'. Comments about thinking and acting differently are part of learning within a team's 'creative zone'. Comments about patients fall into a third learning zone called 'service improvement'. Two golden threads weave their way through the conversations. They are:

- learning through self-organised reflective sessions; and
- learning through reflections on what staff and patients feel, think and do.

In general this nursing team might be described as *disciplined people*, engaging in *disciplined thinking* and *disciplined action* (see Part Three). It might also be described as a healthy team. Also they are not just a collection of individuals, but individuals with particular skills and qualities, interacting in particular ways. It is not (to draw upon Belbin's 1982, team roles work) made up of say, a process manager (ability to chair meetings), a concept developer (visionary), a harmoniser (supporting), critic, technical expert (specialised know-how) and the like. It is the blend within teams that counts. Rust *et al.* (2003) and their Orpheus TPQ approach talk about 'blending'. It was originally developed on what they called the big five model of 'fellowship', 'authority', 'conformity', 'emotion' and 'detail'. Within each, there are extremes, which can be represented thus:

- Fellowship: social skills vs. task focus.
- Authority: tenacity/drive vs. empathy/team skills.
- Conformity: following rules vs. change champion.
- Emotion: sensitive/cautious vs. calm/decisive.
- Detail: eye for detail vs. big picture.

Rust *et al.* (2003) are asking a serious question about what blend of knowledge, skills and sensitivities makes teams work best, in certain situations and work environments. They also open up the possibility that 'positively diverse' team characteristics can lead to highly successful team performance. I will return to the important issue of team diversity later. Doris and the district nursing team seem to have both diversity and togetherness! They have tenacity and empathy. They follow but also make the rules. They can be cautious but also decisive and so on. There is Little Whirlwind, Sunshine, Wise Owl, Little Lamb, Racehorse and of course Doris herself. Between them they create a sense of spirit and teamness. Doris has an eye on the bigger picture, while others are keeping watch on specifics. They participate in certain kinds of knowledge-enabling activities (regular sessions of reflection) that promote constructive and helpful relations between team members and their patients.

TA²LK's three serious questions

Developing reflective healthcare teams that are able to sustain high quality, personalised care has three basic dimensions to it (Fig 18.1). They are:

- the organisation;
- the team; and
- the individual.

It is necessary to recognise that conditions in one dimension critically affect conditions in other dimensions and that for effective team development every dimension needs to be addressed (Stott & Walker 1995). Figure 18.1 shows how **TA²LK** uses three serious questions to tackle these dimensions holistically. They are questions that can be asked by individuals, within teams and across healthcare organisations. At the heart of the process are iterative cycles of reflection and action arising from this.

TA²LK is a very action-oriented, practical improvement process. Getting the most from it requires certain kinds of disciplined thinking and action. Trained **TA²LK** facilitators can help teams with this. The actions are set out in Fig. 18.2. Action arising from STEPs, SURE and ASK is partly based upon staff (and service users where appropriate) consenting to complete short questionnaires. With the use of modern technology, data are computerised by IRP-UK staff and fed back to teams in graphical (portrait) form. Questionnaires are completed anonymously. With recent changes in research governance guidelines, some care needs to be taken with their administration. Some organisations see their use as 'research', others as 'clinical audit'. The former

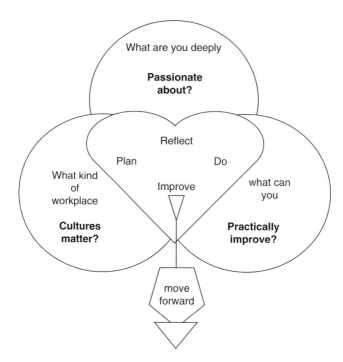

Fig 18.1   TA²LK's three serious questions.

always requires ethical approval. The latter does not. What action to take usually comes from responses to these three questions:

1   Is their use principally to try to improve the quality of patient care in the local setting?
2   Will they involve measuring practice against standards?
3   Do they involve anything being done to patients that would not have been part of their normal routine management?

Normally if the answer is 'yes' to the first two questions and 'no' to the third, it is safe to say that their use conforms to the requirements of clinical audit. With a different pattern of responses, their use may be regarded as research. It is prudent to get in touch with the Central Office for Research Ethics Committees (in the UK) to clarify if research ethics committee approval is needed.

- *STEPs* is action by staff that arises from learning about, 'what it's like to work here, doing my job, with those I work with' (see Fig. 18.3). It comprises three zones. The care, creative and the service improvement zones. In this part of the book, STEPs is described in some detail to illuminate many of the facets of the **TA²LK** process. STEPs makes team (and workplace) cultures concrete. Cultures are the single most pervasive influence on the quality of workplace action. STEPs has been influenced by the literatures described above and developed

Table 18.1 TA²LK and development in three basic dimensions.

The individual	The team	The organisation
Gives staff a picture of what they feel it's like to work where they do, doing what they do, with the people they work with.	Benchmarks team working. Benchmarks the service user's experience.	Benchmarks the performance of teams within/ across disciplines, departments, directorates, etc.
Gives them a picture of how far they feel able to think and act creatively.	Provides a way for teams to assess their learning needs.	Links team performance with service user views.
Gives them a picture of how their 'users' feel about their service.	Benchmarks feelings of team empowerment.	Enables staff to manage their talent effectively and efficiently.
Benchmarks their work. Provides a way to improve individual practice	Gives teams a picture of how far the team feels cohesive, supported, innovative, well led and influential. Provides evidence of organisational responses to major policy drivers. Provides evidence about how far members feel they can trust each other. Identifies problems with communication, decision-making and work pressure. Helps teams make positive choices and decisions.	Supports preparations for service reviews and inspections. Identifies root causes of stress, recruitment and retention problems. Clearly identifies why teams and services are successful.

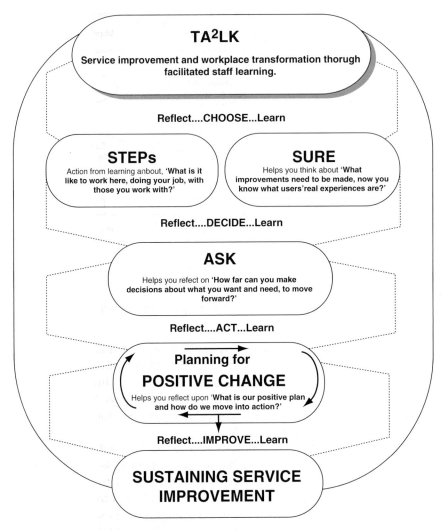

Fig 18.2   TA²LK... its key parts.

by an iterative process of revision and respondent revalidation since 1995. Currently STEPs is a 50-statement (item) questionnaire. All statements have been derived from actual staff comments. Statements have a high face validity. The attributes internal scale reliabilities (Cronbach's alpha) fall within acceptable limits and vary between 0.71 to 0.83. The very latest version of STEPs, at the time of going to press, has been used with 753 teams in health and social care in the UK. STEPs can be used repeatedly as part of a benchmarking process.

- *SURE* enables staff to think about: What improvements need to be made, now we know what our service users' real experiences are? SURE has been developed from an extensive item bank of service user comments gathered in the course of normal practice, over a 5-year

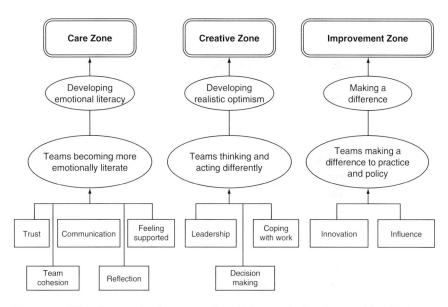

Fig 18.3   The five main features of staff 'portraits' generated by STEPs.

period. It has been progressively revised and revalidated through an iterative process of respondent validation. SURE can be used repeatedly with particular service user groups, or to illuminate specific episodes of care, as part of a benchmarking process. SURE comes in a generic form and specially customised versions for maternity and children's services for example.

- *ASK* invites staff to get themselves organised for action so they can move forward. The question that triggers this process is: How far can you make decisions about what you want and need, to move forward? The ASK part of the **TA²LK** process offers choices to staff. They are invited to make decisions about how they wish to sustain their engagement in the process. No blueprint is offered. Staff are not 'force-fitted' into some kind of pre-specified mould. Staff self-organise for learning through reflection.
- *Planning for POSITIVE CHANGE* brings thinking, people and action together. Those involved are asked: What is your positive plan and how do you move into positive action?
- *SUSTAINING SERVICE IMPROVEMENT* is action that enables participants to keep things going in a principled and evidence-based way.

Chapter 19
The 'faces' of TA^{2}LK

Conventionally, models that describe team development are *linear*. Development is essentially a step-by-step, sequential process. They also include life-cycle and stage models. They all describe development as a one-way process. A good example of this is Tuckman's four-stage model (Tuckman 1965), which includes forming, storming, norming and performing stages. Another traditional approach is one where development is associated with team roles (Belbin 1982) and more recently the Robertson-Cooper Limited 'teamable – making your team work' process. Teamable is premised on a view that we all have a certain amount of flexibility around our typical way of contributing to a team. Teamable helps staff do two things. First, to identify preferred team roles. Second, to enable members to take up roles and responsibilities that they would not ordinarily prefer to do and to do so in a flexible manner. Rather caustically, Syer and Connolly (1996) argue that '... the only form of improvement offered by these models is to replace members who fail to show a certain ability with others who appear to have it'.

TA^{2}LK is different from more traditional processes of team development because its focus is on team learning, facilitated through the practices of reflection. It links team development with the team's ability to learn. Learning through sharing, in turn, influences their wellness. Wellness affects how far teams are able to influence change and respond positively to it. TA^{2}LK is also a social process and needs to be supported within *communities of participation*. These communities can be understood as patterns of action and interaction. Patterns are initiated, terminated and sustained within a socio-cultural and politico-economic context. This context affects what is felt, said and done. TA^{2}LK prioritises the processes of reflection-for-learning and learning-for-improvement. It positions itself socially and politically with the collective, namely the team, who, when sufficiently well organised for learning, can often play a significant part in sustaining service improvement.

The TA^{2}LK process is more holistic, realistic and relevant to service improvement than these linear models. It has been specifically informed, for example, by the work of Kur (1996) and his use of 'face' as a metaphor for team development. The basic idea behind Kur's work is that of teams having 'faces'. At one time a team may wear one face and at another time wear a different face. Each face is associated with certain patterns of relationships and action. The pattern is not linear but more complex. Any face may precede or follow any other face. Teams might move back and forth presenting and then discarding faces according to the exigencies of the moment. Kur describes a total of five faces. Two of them are particularly relevant to this book. They are his descriptions of a team's informing and performing faces. For example when teams wear an informing face, '... their members strive to understand, learn, evaluate and develop a shared mindset... Informing is about coming to grips with shared values... some teams do not engage in these learning processes until well into the life of the team, if at all' (Kur 1996, p. 26). Healthy teams need to embrace and return to their informing face from time to time. The different demands of working life may require this.

In strengthening teams for high performance, Kur argues that we should try to develop conditions to enable teams to wear their performing face as frequently and as continuously as possible. **TA²LK** does just this by ensuring that the reflective process helps teams learn from their experience and get back to their performing face when appropriate. Kur describes a team's performing face in terms of high trust, esprit, openness with one another, role flexibility, active listening and actively seeking ideas from each other. Additionally, decision-making is shared and '... any member of the team may act on behalf of the entire team in the confidence that his or her team-mates will support any action taken'. (Kur 1996, p. 26). A team needing or wanting to change its face is a liberating way to view team development. Changing faces, in any direction, needs to be accepted as normal and responsive to the different demands of practice. **TA²LK** acknowledges this and emphasises that each change creates new learning opportunities. If changes in face are a normal and natural thing, we need a process of team development that describes both the linearity and the ocillarity (back-and-forth) nature of team development (see Fig. 28.1). To reach and sustain high performance, teams need to have the courage, clarity of thinking, agility, political acuity and resilience to get back in touch with the elements in their care and/or creative zones and then move back to their performing face (and elements in their 'service improvement zone') as and when appropriate. Through **TA²LK** a team's current 'face' is reflected back to them, in the form of computer generated 'portraits' (see Fig. 19.1).

TA²LK, team wellness and health

TA²LK has also been specifically informed by the work of Groesbeck and van Aken (2001) and the notion of team wellness. Wellness incorporates two interrelated processes called monitoring and maintenance.

1   *Monitoring* = diagnosing the current state of team working. There are two aspects to monitoring. They are: (a) Taskworking. This is about getting the job done and the knowledge, skills and attitudes needed for this. It is about a team's wellness to perform team tasks. (b) Team-

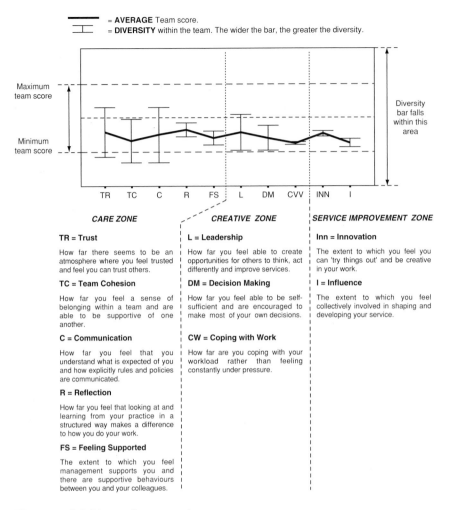

────── = **AVERAGE** Team score.
⊥ = **DIVERSITY** within the team. The wider the bar, the greater the diversity.

Maximum team score

Minimum team score

Diversity bar falls within this area

TR   TC   C   R   FS   L   DM   CVV   INN   I

CARE ZONE   CREATIVE ZONE   SERVICE IMPROVEMENT ZONE

TR = Trust

How far there seems to be an atmosphere where you feel trusted and feel you can trust others.

TC = Team Cohesion

How far you feel a sense of belonging within a team and are able to be supportive of one another.

C = Communication

How far you feel that you understand what is expected of you and how explicitly rules and policies are communicated.

R = Reflection

How far you feel that looking at and learning from your practice in a structured way makes a difference to how you do your work.

FS = Feeling Supported

The extent to which you feel management supports you and there are supportive behaviours between you and your colleagues.

L = Leadership

How far you feel able to create opportunities for others to think, act differently and improve services.

DM = Decision Making

How far you feel able to be self-sufficient and are encouraged to make most of your own decisions.

CW = Coping with Work

How far are you coping with your workload rather than feeling constantly under pressure.

Inn = Innovation

The extent to which you feel you can 'try things out' and be creative in your work.

I = Influence

The extent to which you feel collectively involved in shaping and developing your service.

Fig 19.1   Making cultures real.

working. This is about a team's wellness to work together as a team. Knowledge about other team members (e.g. skill, preferences) sensitivities towards each other (e.g. being respectful) and patterns of interaction (e.g. who supports whom) are all parts of this.

2   *Maintenance* = assuring teams self-generate, self-organise or receive appropriate support that enables them to work and learn together and perform team tasks. ASK contributes an evidence base for this.

Questionnaire data from staff and service users are fed back as computer generated portraits in a way to promote an *appreciative conversation* among participants. The portraits reflect a team's current 'face' and are a catalyst for a conversation about how well the face looks! Each teams' portrait is different. Portraits also change over time.

Staff portrait's have five main features. These are:

1   Attributes in a 'care zone'. This is about a team's *emotional literacy* (Mayer & Salovey 1993, Ashforth & Humphrey 1995, Bar-On *et al.* 2000, Fisher & Ashkanasy 2000, Ashkanasy *et al.* 2002, Freshman & Rubino 2002, Vitello-Cicciu 2002). Development in this zone focuse-son five areas (see Table 22.1). Developing emotional literacy is about-staff being able to transform threat (from change) into the challenge of improvement. To do this a team has to manage its emotions, skilfully.
2   Attributes in a 'creative zone'. This is about *realistic optimism*. Development in this zone focuses on three areas (see Table 23.1). Developing realistic optimism involves thinking and acting differently. To do this a team has to manage its ability to be creative, skilfully.
3   Attributes in a 'service improvement zone'. This is about a team's ability to *make a difference* to health service practice and policy. Development in this zone focuses on two areas (see Table 11). Making a difference is about the team's ability to manage their impact, skilfully.
4   A solid (blue wavy) line that depicts a team's mean score for each attribute in each zone. Participants are encouraged (sometimes by an external facilitator) to reflect on the line's general shape and form, as well as on points that are relatively high and low.
5   A (pink) bar that shows the degree of diversity of view, amongst staff, for each attribute in each zone. The solid line (average score for each attribute) masks any diversity of view, within a team. To illuminate this, a 'diversity within the team' bar is shown. The wider the bar, the greater the diversity of view. The width of the bar represents diversity around the mean. The eye should focus on the width of each bar, around each point in the portrait and between zones.

These portraits are processed by IRP-UK and fed back to staff with an invitation for teams to 'put their own story to their own portrait'. The conversation that ensues is usually supported by a trained **TA²LK** facilitator. Staff are encouraged to respond to the following:

1   From STEPs the most satisfying thing to us is …
2   From STEPs the most surprising thing to us is …
3   From STEPs the most worrying thing to us is …

To enrich and deepen some of these reflective conversations, teams use a version of root cause analysis (RCA) to 'get behind' their line and bar. Reflecting on root causes is important because it means asking what, how and why questions. It is a learning process that helps teams get to the root causes that give rise to the shape of the line and the width of each bar. The aim of RCA is not to blame, but to learn how to sustain what is good in the portrait and improve those things that the team are less happy about.

In Fig. 19.1 the solid line (average team score for each attribute) is fairly depressed in each of the three zones. No point rises above the mid-line. This portrait represents a *team in poor health*. The lowest points on the portrait show that team members are not *coping with work*, do not feel *influential* and are not experiencing a feeling of *team cohesion*. Other parts of the line serve to reinforce a view that this team is not in a good state of health and well-being. When attention shifts to a consideration of the width of each bar, the team's wellness to perform tasks and work together also appears to be problematic. We can see there is very little consensus in the care zone. This means that initial team development efforts might usefully be targeted here as emotional literacy is the fundamental building block for improving team performance. The position of the line and width of the bars in the service improvement zone, suggest that members of this team do not feel innovative or influential. There is a consensus over these views.

The most important thing about feeding back the STEPs (and SURE) portraits to teams, is that *it is staff themselves who interpret their own portrait/s. They put their own story to their own line and bars.* This makes learning more meaningful and signals to staff that they need to take some responsibility for their own learning. The ownership of the improvement process rests with the team. The portrait acts as a benchmark against which future team working and learning can be measured. Conversations of possibility are a precursor for building a positive plan for change.

Chapter 20

TA²LK as a facilitated team learning process

The primary aim of facilitation is, 'to enable participants to develop into a self-managing, self-regulating and self-monitoring team able to provide and sustain high quality, personalised care'. Normally teams have some help, from appropriately trained **TA²LK** facilitators, to 'make a good start' with the process. Usually this is three to four two-hour sessions. Facilitation is a challenging endeavour. Training as a certified **TA²LK** facilitator normally takes 5 days (equivalent) staff time and involves becoming skilful at *looking for learning*. To help with this, facilitators are encouraged to use simple, but powerful, learning frameworks to help them (and all participants) look for learning. Two examples of this are given in Table 20.1. One uses the de Bono 'PMI' process. The other a 'PPC' framework.

Everyone learns differently (see Starting Points: Through the Learning Lens). Facilitators have to work out the 'best' way to enable participants to learn together. This involves them understanding what helps and can hinder learning. For example:

- The differences between groups and teams.
- Team membership issues.
- Team building strategies.
- Group dynamics: motives, (hidden) agendas, expectations, competitiveness, power struggles, isolation, alienation, anger, fear, grief, sharing uncertainties, rewards, praise, belonging.
- How to work with anxiety. Acceptance anxiety: will/am I accepted, liked, wanted? Orientation anxiety: will I understand what's going on? Performance anxiety: will I be able to make a contribution, be competent, control the situation to meet my needs?
- How to enable teams to move from safe to personal responses by working with defensiveness. Submission: withdrawal, shut-down, powerlessness, loss of identity. Flight: irrelevant talk, joking, gossip about trivialities, becoming a pair that breaks away from the group. Attack: facilitator is resisted, their suggestions rejected, relevance or competence challenged, others scape-goated, blamed.
- The characteristics of effective and high performing teams and how to enable them to get there.

TA²LK facilitator training also involves enabling participants to reflect on their espoused values and values-in-action (see Part Two). It gives facilitators the skills and confidence to invite participants to explore:

Table 20.1   TA²LK and looking for learning.

1. The P.M.I. framework

→ **P = Plus Points**	Things you felt were particularly good and worthy about what you saw and heard.
→**M = Minus Points**	Things you felt didn't quite work and could be a further source of reflection and possible improvement.
→**I = Interesting Points**	Things that particularly interested you, surprised, intrigued, puzzled you.

2. The P.P.C. framework

→**P = Positive**	Facilitators try to comment first and favourably on things that were particularly good/praiseworthy. No matter how 'bad' or difficult the conversation was for staff (and/or them), they try to find something positive to say … and mean it!
→**P = Possibilities**	Facilitators engage in a reflective conversation about the possibilities for extending participant ideas, revising them, taking them forward, making greater sense of them, etc. Facilitators try to help to reframe and move thinking and actions forward where appropriate. It's about exploring personal and collective actions, professional and political possibilities.
→**C = Concerns**	Facilitators try to enable participants to state these constructively and honestly. Timing is crucial. Giving space to respond to concerns is critical. Space to review/reflect/reconsider. Facilitators try to use phrases like, 'I have a concern about … Could you help me understand how you might address this?

- *Values Clarification.* Where do participants agree? Why do they agree over these things?
- *Value Conflicts.* Where do participants disagree? Why do they disagree over these things?
- *Value Consensus.* What does 'improving practice' mean for participants?

Facilitation training also involves building confidence to 'sense' and 'seize' the moment to enable participants to end the reflective meeting ethically. This involves embracing two kinds of reflection.

- *Reflection-for-Understanding.* What do we feel we have learnt? What do we now know?
- *Reflection-for-Improvement.* What is our next step? How might we try to improve things?

Facilitation and overcoming resistance

Staff may have many reasons for resisting change. They may simply be change-weary. Resistance might be borne out of anxiety. It may be due to a conflict of values. 'Resistance is a way of saying "no" to change. Wisely used, this is a valuable contribution to the change process. Randomly or irresponsibly employed, it causes unbearable stress and considerable bad feeling' (O'Connor 1993, p. 25). With each improvement effort there are impediments. Resistance is the most obvious barrier. Resistance can be either intentional or unintentional. It can be covert or overt. It can develop almost without warning, or we can see it brewing for quite a while, before it actually comes to a head.

O'Connor (1993) suggests that our first move should be to discover the nature and force of the resistance and then we should explore what causes it. He developed a matrix that helps us understand the different types of resistance that might be encountered in an improvement process (see Fig. 20.1).

Covert resistance

This is where support for improvement is either concealed or undefined. In some teams, a covert resister operates secretly, undermining improvement efforts if such efforts are felt to work against their own vested interests. Covert resistance is serious.

Overt resistance

This type of resister expresses a point of view openly and offers reasons for disagreement. Overt resistance can lead to a healthy debate and perhaps some overt conflict that needs to be handled sensitively.

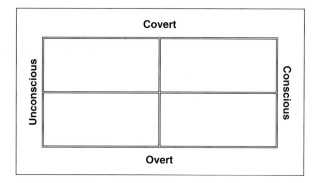

Fig 20.1   Four basic types of resistance (after O'Connor 1993).

Unconscious resistance

This is a tricky one to handle because team members who behave in this way are often unaware that they are indeed resisting improvement efforts. They may feel that they are 'innocent' and just doing their job.

Conscious resistance

This kind of resistance can also be highly problematic. People often take up this posture after careful consideration of the options and alternatives before them. They may be misinformed or even self-serving. However, their opinions need to be aired and debated.

O'Connor goes on to elaborate on these four extremes of resistance, coming up with four caricatures or types of resister (Fig. 20.2).

Covert and unconscious: the survivor

These resisters do not realise they are undermining change. They often do not know they are failing to meet team commitments and tasks or even understand the implications of their behaviours. Their activities are largely undetected because higher profile or more urgent team work screens or masks them. They simply soldier on, getting the job done in the way they know how to do it. When their lack of adaptation to change is discovered, they are as surprised and disappointed as anyone in the team. They often believe they are doing a good job, and feel discouraged by the wasted effort.

Covert and conscious: the saboteur

These resisters undermine improvement efforts within the team, while pretending to support them. Some saboteurs are motivated simply by a wish to minimise disruption and discomfort. They believe that by verbally supporting the change and doing nothing, the initiative will go away. However, others have a more sinister motive. These individuals

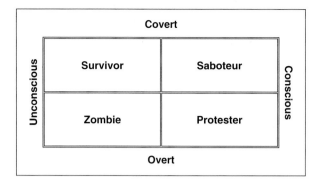

Fig 20.2 Four kinds of resister (after O'Connor 1993).

intend to sabotage team improvement plans for their own gain. While this is a far less frequent occurrence than the tactic of ignoring responsibility, it is a strong possibility within highly competitive teams and in demanding healthcare settings.

Overt and unconscious: the zombie

These resisters are an extreme case of the survivor. They are so accustomed to acting in a certain way that they seem unable to change. While they verbally agree to do whatever is asked of them, they have neither the will nor the ability to create the change. Gradually and openly, they revert to their former patterns of behaviour. While they realise that they are not doing what they agreed to do, they mysteriously do not regard this as resistance. They are simply avoiding the change until they are reminded once again that they must alter their behaviour.

Overt and conscious: the protestor

One name that some might give to these staff would be a 'pain in the neck'. Protestors never seem to rest in pointing out the failings of a proposed improvement effort. Their protests can be very principled ones. On the positive side, these team member's protests can help as a reality check. They can discourage rash or sudden decisions being made. They can work to stop teams getting carried away in the euphoria of the moment. On balance, protestors are the most visible and for some, the most interesting kind of resisters that need managing skilfully. Their resistance is not only open, but they are able to discuss their position clearly and often rationally.

Developing reflective facilitators for reflective teams

TA²LK holds a belief that it is reflective facilitators that are best placed to develop reflective teams. What follows are eight qualities facilitators are helped to develop. Facilitators are given a portfolio in which to record their responses to each question, inside each quality. Questions are answered with particular teams in mind.

Quality 1.   Learning culture
How far have you created a context for participants to focus on learning about practice and learning for the improvement of practice?

Quality 2.   Making learning visible
How far have you been able to make explicit the values (hopes, motivations, beliefs) that guide participant work and what helps/hinders the process of putting values-into-action?

Quality 3.   Working with uncertainty
How far have you been able to be flexible and responsive to participant needs and views as they arise?

Quality 4.   Participant decision-making
·How far have you been able to facilitate participant decision-making through knowledge/sharing information?

Quality 5.   Valuing diversity
How far have you recognised individual gifts and talents and provided opportunities for individuals to non/participate?

Quality 6.   Momentum
How far have you enabled participants to experience and talk about moving their practice and policies forward?

Quality 7.   Improvement
How far have you enabled participants to share and acknowledge evidence of improvement in: What they think? What they say (e.g. being more influential)? What they do (e.g. their practice)? Where they work?

Quality 8.   Reflection
How far have you enabled participants to learn through structured, supported and regular reflection-on-practice?

Chapter 21

Cultures of care

Caring for each other, together with a range of knowledge-enabling processes, is the solid foundation upon which a reflective team's work is based. Most staff opt to tackle the attributes in the 'care zone' first. Fig. 21.1 shows that there can be high levels of care amongst staff in a team, characterised by *sharing* and feelings of *connectedness*. These attributes are missing with low levels of care. Here *individualism* and *contrived collegiality* are more prevalent. When care is high, teams work well due to a process of knowledge and skill sharing. These are given and received. The sharing of what is felt and known becomes a basis for risk taking, innovation and better practice. This is subject to both peer critique and celebration. Teams learn well when there is a connectedness between members. This does not just mean a 'physical' connection through face-to-face encounters. It is not only about regular team meetings and stable team membership as these are often hard to sustain. It is a connectedness arising from shared values and a clearly articulated response to the statement, 'this is what we stand for'. Connectedness is felt when members are together but also when they are apart.

Sharing and connectedness are predicated upon establishing and sustaining five key team attributes. These are:

1 (creating and sustaining) trust;
2 (building) team cohesion;
3 (meaningful) communication; and
4 (supporting) each other.

All these processes are nourished and fuelled by the practices of reflection. Taken together they contribute to a team's *Emotional Literacy*. A team's STEPs portrait shows their state of emotional literacy. This is also a reflection of their state of wellness.

Reflective teams as emotionally literate teams

Greater team working and more emphasis on workplace learning in the NHS, will soon translate into greater demand for staff with high levels of emotional intelligence and literacy (Weisinger 1998, Cherniss & Goleman 2001). The **TA²LK** process enables teams to develop their emotional literacy. This is defined as a team member's ability to use the practices of reflection to, 'understand their own and other member's emotional

Team wellness			
		(Team) Working	*(Team) Learning*
Cultures of care ↑ ↓	Low care	• No active empathy with other members • Lone worker mindset **INDIVIDUALISM** • Expects little from colleagues, receives little • Unshared certainty	• Give and take approach • Information exchanged **CONTRIVED COLLEGIALITY** • Defence and blame • No mutual dependence
	High care	• Genuine interest in what each other does • Members receive emotional support **SHARING** • Access to expertise and ideas • Knowledge and skill sharing	• Members 'live with' decisions jointly made • Work through practice issues together **CONNECTEDNESS** • Joint commitment to practice improvement • Passionately reason with each other

Fig 21.1   Some links between 'cultures of care' and team wellness.

states, to positively express and manage their own emotions and respond to the emotions of others, in ways that enable members of the team to monitor and maintain a good sense of team wellness'.

Weare (2004) suggests that there are three broad areas of competence that comprise emotional literacy. All these are related to a longstanding interest in the practices of reflection, namely that of 'being-human-well' (see Part Two). The areas are:

1   self-understanding;
2   understanding, expressing and managing emotions; and
3   understanding social situations and making relationships.

How can we care for others if we cannot care for ourselves? Developing in area 1 is a good start. It is made up of a clear, positive and realistic self-concept, having a sense of optimism and experiencing a sense of coherence. Weare (2004) refers to *self-concept* as including:

• Liking ourselves, even though we may not always like our behaviours.
• Valuing and respecting ourselves as unique individuals.
• Being able to identify and feel positive about our own strengths.
• Being able to identify our own limitations and vulnerabilities, and accepting them without undue self-blame or guilt.

A *sense of optimism* means, for example, believing:

• That the problems and difficulties we may be experiencing are a challenge not a barrier.
• That we have the potential to succeed in the things we want to.
• That when things go wrong it is not necessarily our own fault.

- That we can and will change the things about ourselves that we do not like, that are under our control.

Feeling a *sense of coherence* involves things like:

- Making sense of our multiple selves.
- Seeing the world as meaningful, and events as comprehensible and connected together.

Weare (2004) describes the elements of area 2 thus. It comprises:

- *Experiencing a full range of emotions* (e.g. talking openly and accurately about our emotions, including naming the full range of emotions).
- *Understanding the causes of our emotions* (e.g. being aware of the extent to which our emotions are triggered by factors 'out there' or 'in here').
- *Expressing emotion* (e.g. expressing our emotions to ourselves, feeling the anger or the sadness, crying, letting off steam in a safe way).
- *Managing our responses to our emotions* (e.g. expressing our difficult emotions appropriately, including safe expression of anger or sorrow).
- *Increasing our emotional pleasure* (e.g. being aware of what aspects of our lives generate pleasurable emotions).
- *Using information about our emotions to plan and solve problems* (e.g. being creative and seeing several ways through and round a problem).
- *Resilience and determination* (e.g. learning from a difficult experience and using it to aid our own development).

The components of Weare's third area of understanding social situations and making relationships are about:

- *Attachment and bonding* (e.g. trusting others to meet your needs, love and care about you).
- *Empathy* (e.g. sensitivity, being able to intuit how people are feeling from their tone and body language).
- *Communication* (e.g. listening actively to others in ways that encourage them to talk and to feel understood.
- *Managing relationships* (e.g. establishing appropriate levels of trust with others, for example by being authentic and reliable, knowing how much to disclose and to whom about ourselves, and how to keep confidences about others.
- *Autonomy* (e.g. thinking for yourself and taking action consistent with your beliefs and principles).

All of these areas are worthy of development. They are not mutually exclusive. Arguably, team development is predicated upon individual competence in areas 1 and 2. STEPs focuses particularly on developing a team's emotional literacy in area 3. In essence the 'care zone' is about enabling teams to create inter-personal warmth, togetherness and a platform to talk-to-learn.

Chapter 22

The Care Zone: developing a team's emotional literacy

Reflective teams are emotionally literate ones. There are five attributes in the care zone that can be a focus for attention and development. They are shown in Table 22.1. Staff make a tick-in-the-box response, mostly true/mostly false, to each of the items in the questionnaire.

Trusting me, trusting you: an essential building block for developing a reflective team

Recently I was asked to work with a team in orthopaedics from a large district general hospital. We were discussing how far their existing process of working together and the 'ground rules' for this, were as they would wish it to be and what they were getting out of it. Some felt the team was fragmenting and things were 'not like they were', due to the constant pressures from service reviews and re-organisation. We soon began to talk about 'trust'. I invited them to peel back the layers of meaning behind their use of the word. We explored two dimensions of trust. First, what an 'atmosphere' of trust felt like within the team. Second, what trusting behaviours looked like as they worked together and with their patients. We began with a focus on the words they associated with trust. After much discussion, the following appeared on a series of flip chart papers: openness, honesty, fairness, keeping promises, loyalty, consistency of behaviour, mutual confidence in each other and being available. It soon became obvious that these meant quite different things to each member of staff. To explore them further the team began to work in pairs and to make something, with coloured card, which illustrated aspects of two of the dimensions of trust, those stated above. To enable them to do this in the time available, the team was offered as a catalyst for reflection and action, an expression of trust in the shape of a wheel. In the wheel were five words. We talked about these and how they might impact on their team work and learning. The basic wheel is shown in Fig. 22.1.

The wheel was made of large pieces of card that staff could handle and pass between them. It helped make the discussion concrete. Members were asked to pick up a piece of their choice and express what it meant to them. We then explored the links between parts of the wheel. For example, between words and actions. That is between what staff say (to each other) and what they do (together). Between what staff do (actions)

Table 22.1 Attributes of the care zone.

Attribute	Description
Trust	How far there seems to be an atmosphere where you feel trusted and feel you can trust others. *Sample item: I feel I can trust the people I work with.*
Team Cohesion	How far you feel a sense of belonging within a team and are able to be supportive of one another. *Sample item: I feel a sense of togetherness with others.*
Communication	How far you feel that you understand what is expected of you and how explicitly rules and policies are communicated. *Sample item: We usually get to know things after they've already happened.*
Reflection	How far you feel that looking at and learning from your practice, in a structured way, makes a difference to how you do your work. *Sample item: Reflection helps me see my work in new and different ways.*
Feeling Supported	The extent to which you feel management supports you and there are supportive behaviours between you and your colleagues. *Sample item: I feel that my manager really stands up for us.*

and why (motives). All of these expressions helped deepen the team's collective appreciation of the centrality of trust in team working and learning and the challenges to sustaining it.

For the next hour, pairs of staff worked on making their wheels. Then they were invited to work in fours, sharing their accomplishments, exploring points of connection and diversity. One wheel, which the team felt was particularly helpful and that might be a basis for moving forward for them, is the one shown in Fig. 22.2.

Their wheel reflects an important number of inter-dependencies. For example, between trust and a recognition that members had personal and professional issues to deal with. Between trust and their perceived ability to work together, trust and supporting each other, and so on. What we have in this wheel are some fundamental prerequisites for reflective team working and learning. It begins to point the way to understanding what reflective teams are like, need and do. In terms of a culture of care

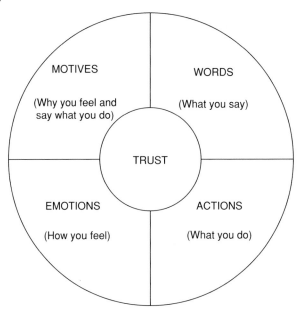

Fig 22.1   A trust wheel: a catalyst for thinking and acting differently.

(sharing and connectedness) we can sense that trust, support, communication and working together (often referred to as a sense of team cohesion) are important. The metaphor of a wheel was used because the team were feeling that things were 'not like they were'. The wheels were coming off the team bus, or were certainly wobbling! A wheel conveyed a little of the dynamics of building and sustaining trust. It suggested that teams often get stuck and may even feel they are going backwards, when fundamental attributes like trust begin to be put under pressure. Although the idea of a wheel is rather mechanical and other metaphors might be more appropriate, it was helpful in this particular context of reflecting on team working and learning. It was important to explore with staff how they might keep their wheel turning and moving forward.

Trust within teams

Trust is one particular attribute, in STEPs, that participants are invited to reflect upon. Trust and mutual dependency need to be part of team life and embedded in policy statements and strategic plans. But this might be problematic. In a provocative article by Harrison (2003), he asks the question 'What has actually been happening in New Labour's NHS?' He identifies three trends, namely increasing managerialism, a very strong trend of regulation and, closely related to regulation, increasing technocracy. By this he means that in any given circumstance there is a single correct way of doing things. He develops his argument in relation

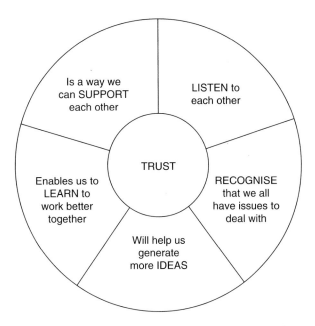

Fig 22.2 Our trust wheel: an orthopaedic team.

to evidence-based practice and policy. With regard to regulation, he says, 'Ministers and indeed top managers, are traditionally rather fond of reorganising: it shuffles the spoils around and is something they can be confident of achieving. While organisation is important, a strong theme running through many of these changes is that of low levels of trust. People cannot be trusted to get on with their jobs adequately, so they and their organisations need to be controlled by rules and constantly inspected. Some people are indeed not to be trusted, as evidenced by the recent succession of NHS scandals, but more regulation and control only results in a reluctance to blow the whistle and a damaging professional culture of live and let live' (Harrison, 2003, p. 3). It is interesting to note that when Lord Hunt of Kings Heath was junior health minister for New Labour, he reported (Hunt, 2003) that the most difficult question asked of him, by NHS staff was, 'Why don't you trust us?' So who is able to trust whom? Where is it best to place our trust? How are we able to make this judgement?

Positive expectations and the willingness to become vulnerable are critical elements in any definition of trust (Costa *et al.* 2001). The former point is about having positive expectations of others. The latter point is often translated into a willingness to rely on others. Most views of trust are related to individual attributions about other people's intentions and motives, which underlie their behaviour. **TA²LK** helps develop trust in teams by enabling participants to explore their:

- *Propensity to trust.* This is a willingness of staff to trust others. This varies between individuals and teams. People differ in their propensity to trust. Who we are working with, on what task and where, all affect our propensity to trust another. This is further put under pressure when staff find themselves in unfamiliar situations, doing tasks they might feel less confident doing and with others that challenge them. This is relevant to both staff–staff and staff–user relationships.
- *Perceived trustworthiness.* This makes a crucial contribution to processes of knowledge-sharing and feelings of connectedness in teams. It is about how individual team members expect others to be and to behave and is related to things like our perceptions of the person's character, intentions, actions and the congruence between what staff say and do. Sometimes staff perceptions are conditioned by the media, someone's reputation, status and disciplinary background.
- *Trusting behaviours.* This is about the willingness to be vulnerable to others whose actions staff do not control. A tricky one. Trust is undermined in teams when there is not an overt behavioural congruence between what staff say and do. In cases of incongruence we can get distrust, cover-ups, blame, denial and the like. Lower levels of trust are co-related with a tendency to share less information and ideas. So team members feel less connected.

Chapter 23

The Creative Zone: developing a team's ability to think and act differently

The 'care zone' focused on *emotional literacy* and team member's developmental action in five areas (see Table 7). A developing emotional literacy was about staff being able to transform threat (from change) into the challenge of improvement. To do this a team had to manage its emotions, skilfully. The 'creative zone' focuses on *realistic optimism*, which involves thinking and acting differently. To do this a team has to manage its ability to be creative, skilfully. A developmental starting point is the way staff are able to 'see' and talk about their worlds of work 'as they are', but also develop the mental energy to act positively towards a desired improvement. In gathering data for this book, it has become apparent that a team's capacity to stay appropriately focused and realistically optimistic is about developmental action in three areas. These are shown in Table 23.1. A team's performance, member health and happiness are dependent upon the way staff reflect upon the attributes in the creative zone (Gladwell 2002, Kluska *et al.* 2004, Parker & Morris 2004, Richards 2004). Development requires some positive thinking. Negative staff thoughts are also important as they help direct our attention to needs that are not currently being met.

In this section of the book I want to elaborate upon two of the attributes in the zone. One is receiving much attention in the UK's National Health Service. It is leadership (Snow 2001, French 2004, Donnor & Wheeler 2004, Herbert & Edgar 2004). The other is a significant blind spot. It is the interplay between creativity, coping with work and recovery.

Effective leadership

There is of course a vast literature about leaders and leadership and a great deal of interest and investment currently in it in UK health and social care. In the context of more team-based work cultures, what kind of leaders should we be trying to nurture and support? Second, given the emphasis on a 'modern NHS' and so presumably the development of 'modern teams', what might be the personality and behaviours of 'modern leaders' for these modern teams? Third, given a target and performance-driven health service, what kind of leadership really matters? In a very interesting book by Sashkin and Sashkin (2003) 'transformational' leadership is examined because they feel this is a kind of leadership that matters. Their central argument is that this type of

Table 23.1 Attributes of the creative zone.

Attribute	Description
Leadership	How far you feel able to create opportunities for others to think, act differently and improve services. *Sample item: I take a stand on difficult work issues.*
Decision Making	How far you feel able to be self-sufficient and are encouraged to make most of your own decisions. *Sample item: I am confident in the decisions I make.*
Coping With Work	How far you are coping with your workload rather than feeling constantly under pressure. *Sample item: The hours I work are manageable.*

leadership makes a critical difference to performance. They argue that these leaders 'transform' people from dutiful followers into self-directed staff who go beyond simply doing what is expected of them.

TA²LK encourages participants to join up leadership with a team's chosen improvement efforts by:

- *Working through* issues, possibilities and challenges.
- *Working on* improving practice and policy by making small steps.

It encourages participants to *work through* 'big ideas' and *work on* 'small steps'. This means thinking politically, organisationally, culturally and strategically and also thinking methodically, practically, realistically and sensibly. Leadership within a team is crucial for this. A number of trigger questions stimulate conversations of possibility. Examples of eight of them are shown in Table 23.2.

Some realistic optimism in a team's responses to the contents of Table 23.2 often depends upon effective leaders within the team. One source of this may be a team leader. A view of leadership as more 'distributed' means there may be many sources of realistic optimism within a team. When engaging in the **TA²LK** process, Bernhard & Walsh's (1995 pp. 18–23) four key qualities of effective leaders act as a catalyst for reflection and action. The qualities are:

- *Self-awareness*: of strengths and limitations.
- *Assertiveness*: being able to express one's feelings, needs and wants and our ability to fight for what we believe is right for staff and service users.

Table 23.2   Change won't happen by magic.

Reflection on ...	Some trigger questions
Leadership	Where will your inspiration come from?
Resources	How will you get what you need?
Strategies	What's your overall 'game plan'?
Policies and Procedures	What's already 'out there' that's useful to you?
Difference	How will you keep 'chipping away' until your plan makes a difference?
Decisions	How will you know if your plan is moving in the right direction?
Dissemination	How will you keep 'drip-feeding' your achievements to others?
Determination	How will you stay focused on the 'little things' that can make a big difference?

- *Accountability*: being able to justify the positive *and* negative outcomes of our actions.
- *Advocacy*: supporting, defending and maintaining the cause of someone or something.

Staff are then invited to rate themselves for each of these four qualities, on a scale of 1 to 5. They have to explain and justify their scores. In pairs, team members then rate each other. Through a reflective conversation the two ratings are then compared. Eventually this opens up a possibility for a whole team discussion about their perceptions of effective leadership (see Table 23.3).

Leadership and creative care

Leadership influences trust within and between teams and trust informs and transforms leaders and leadership. Let me illuminate some of this complexity. Rogers (1995) suggested that leaders need to apply five fundamental strategies, consistently and repeatedly, to create a high-trust workplace for staff. I have elaborated upon his suggestions thus.

1 *Create a high-trust vision.* This emphasis is upon leaders promoting relationships that enable the achievement of common goals and where staff treat each other with respect and dignity. Organisational cultures where turf-protection, position power and bureaucratic hierarchy rule OK, make this a challenging leadership task.

Table 23.3 Some qualities of effective leaders (after Bernhard & Walsh 1995).

How do you rate yourself?	Poor 1	2	↔ Good 3	4	5
			SCORE		
Self-awareness	□	□	□	□	□
My reason for this score:					
Assertiveness	□	□	□	□	□
My reason for this score:					
Accountability	□	□	□	□	□
My reason for this score:					
Advocacy	□	□	□	□	□
My reason for this score:					

How does your colleague rate you?	Poor 1	2	↔ Good 3	4	5
			SCORE		
Self-awareness	□	□	□	□	□
My reason for this score:					
Assertiveness	□	□	□	□	□
My reason for this score:					
Accountability	□	□	□	□	□
My reason for this score:					
Advocacy	□	□	□	□	□
My reason for this score:					

2 *Know yourself.* Here a leader's ability to be reflexive is crucial. It is about leaders examining their own kinds and levels of trust in others and their own trustworthiness. As I have argued earlier, knowing your own values is an important starting point to understanding your behaviours. Rogers (1995, p. 12) states, *'Leaders need to look at themselves realistically and diagnose where they are demonstrating trust in others and where they are not'.*

3 *Build bridges of communication.* This is tied-up with expressions of honesty and openness. With some teams this is more easily said than done! Good leaders might usefully spend time with their staff exploring what these two words actually mean, in practice. Just how open can we be with others? How honest? When would it be unwise, inappropriate or insensitive to be fully open and honest? Where does whistle-blowing fit with this kind of intention? How does the rhetoric of building open and fair cultures and eradicating blame-free ones articulate with this? Rogers does not raise these issues. What he does say is that leaders can build bridges of communication by showing

respect, letting staff know that they are listening to them, by encouraging their involvement and by sharing their thoughts about working better together.

4   *Encourage team members to trust each other.* This sounds very reasonable but of course is full of particular challenges for particular teams. Leadership becomes a matter of enabling members to trust one another to keep their promises, maintain confidences and support each other. We begin to get a hint of a view of a more self-led, self-organising team here.

5   *Practise what you preach.* This is the obvious exhortation that leaders need to walk-the-talk by, '... *willingly discussing sensitive issues, admitting when they are wrong, expressing their own fears and anxieties and doing more listening and less yelling and telling. The hypocrisy of espousing one behaviour and then exhibiting another is a prescription for disaster in creating an environment where trust becomes the predominant working relationship emotion*' (Rogers 1995, p. 12).

When teams and organisations are in difficulty, it is trust that is needed to fuel any improvement process (DePree 1997). Rather depressingly, Fairholm and Fairholm (2000) and Handy (1996) comment that few organisations can boast about their processes of instilling and encouraging trust in teams and across organisations. In the classic work of Bennis (1993) he expresses a view that positive change requires leaders, first and foremost, to gain team member's trust. They then need to work to express the vision of something being 'better', clearly, so that there is a shared understanding of this and some collective 'buy-in'. Developing individual leaders will not be enough. Communities of leaders are needed especially if the message from the Institute of Medicine (IOM) (2001) report *Crossing the Quality Chasm; a New Health System for the 21st Century* is to be taken seriously. The report sets out six aims for any health system. Briefly, these are care delivered by high-performing healthcare teams that is safe, effective, patient-centred, timely, efficient and equitable. Such an agenda is out of reach if the goals of leadership development are more concerned with individual career enhancement rather than service improvement.

The work of Perryman and Robinson (2003) and Fairholm and Fairholm (2000) takes leadership issues back to an understanding of workplace cultures. The former concentrate more on the quality of working life in the NHS, on working together and how this is crucially related to staff feeling valued and involved. The latter explain how a lack of a trusting culture encourages discord and disharmony, not only in teams, but throughout organisations. Cultures then, more than strategies and structures need to be understood first. Some of the forces they found that contributed to learning-impoverished workplace cultures were poor interpersonal communication, apathy, alienation and self-interest. These were related to the way power was being used, the way status was exercised, perceptions by team members of an 'enemy within', stress and burn-out. Leaders need to reflect on the potency of these forces. Asking questions and not worrying about not knowing the answers, is an important leadership challenge. *'It's not right or even the responsibility of a leader always to have the right answers . . . It is, however, the responsibility of a leader to acknowledge that . . . crucial questions exist for every organisation and every individual within an organisation. . . . Ultimately, struggling together with the critical questions will do more to define a successful organisation than all the answers in the world. In my view, asking the critical questions, in the right ways, at the appropriate times, helps define those who are caring enough to lead'* (Pellicer 2003, pp. 4–5).

Developing reflective teams through 'quiet leaders'

Developing reflective teams appears to be nurtured by a new kind of leaders. I am calling them 'quiet leaders'. They appear to make teams work well. They stimulate and support a culture of reflection within a team. Quiet leaders are not silent. They work in a particular way. Working locally in a 'quiet' manner makes their influence ripple out like the 'butterfly effect' in chaos theory. This can cause major systemic improvements and workplace transformations (Wheatley 1999). There are many kinds of leaders and leadership. The view contained within STEPs is a distributed kind. Not leadership by a 'helmsman', heroine or hero. Not leadership invested in one person. It is a conception that opens up the possibility that a team can have more than one leader, more than one kind of leader and that this is right and proper. A view of a team that has many of its members acting like leaders, subscribes to the belief that there are skills and sensitivities of leadership within all of us. In Dot's district nursing team this is the case. The example is also included to show how Dot has many of the qualities of a quiet leader. In listening to data from 753 health and social care teams the following ten qualities of quiet leaders have emerged.

1 *Quiet leaders are good learners: they change themselves, not just others.* In this sense they are excellent examples of reflective practitioners able to be reflexive and with the will and ability to change their practices and even their fundamental values. They are conscious of and actively work at contradictions in their practice. They actively account for themselves and take a personal interest in working at the interfaces presented earlier between the I/me and us/we. In short they can take charge of their own learning.

2 *Quiet leaders are values-driven: they are concerned about what the team stands for.* It is often said that what staff do or do not know is relatively easy to address. But clarifying and 'living out' what staff articulate as

their values, is a big challenge (Peter 2004). I have found that quiet leaders attend to those things that give staff the reasons for doing what they do. The things that make them the kind of professionals they are. What the team stands for matters to them. What also matters is the way they reflect on two value-laden questions: What do I stand for as a leader? What legacy do I want to leave?

3   *Quiet leaders reflect on patterns of power: they encourage a culture of questioning.* This is very much linked with one of the interests of reflection described in Part Two. It is a way of releasing the team's ability to be creative. Creativity can be both an individual and team activity (Lofy 1998, Ollila 2000, Durant 2002, Fitzgerald *et al.* 2003). It includes skills and aptitudes that make the process of innovation possible. Put another way it is the quiet leader's ability to encourage others to question both the ends and the means in healthcare management and service delivery. These leaders are personally open to challenge and expect other members to be likewise. They quietly allow power to circulate freely within the team. In this clever way, power becomes a pattern of relations, understood by everyone. Members are not trapped or condemned by powerful 'others'. Each is encouraged to incorporate an awareness of the impact of their own power, which may be derived from various sources, (eg. clinical experience, doing a course) on team working and learning. But if power within teams is exchanged and permitted to circulate, then there are always opportunities for resistance.

4   *Quiet leaders are good readers: they want ideas from everywhere.* By good readers I mean they have a kind of emotional and political literacy that enables them to read the professional landscape and spy-out sources of opportunity for the team. They display a personal aesthetic that enables them to make the complexities of service improvement understandable. In their actions, they convey a spirit of the team working to make problems their friends. Because of their other qualities, they do not think that they have all the answers. The minute this happens, learning stops! Quiet leaders let their members know that they want to hear from anyone who has an idea. They celebrate ideas when they are offered. This encourages others to find their voice. In turn it motivates the team to express even more ideas.

5   *Quiet leaders develop 'alongsideness', not leader-follower relationships.* There is much in the literature about individual leaders dreaming up and articulating a vision and motivating (not intimidating) others (followers) to execute it. An important quality of those that lead like this is their ability to let others (team members) know exactly how their efforts are helping staff achieve this vision. But in learning-impoverished NHS workplace cultures things happen to undermine this. For example, team members are afraid to take initiatives and decisions for fear of making a mistake and getting things wrong. In gathering data for this book, quiet leaders do not appear to be locked

into a leader-follower mindset but see team relationships in a very collegial, cooperative and connected way. Because of this, visions are co-constructed, with the team. Achieving the vision is then seen as another part of the team's collective process of becoming. Alongsideness, not as a parallel relationship, but one with connection, will inevitably be seen by some as an expression of power reduction. But in this case, perceptions by some of less, is in reality, more! Pound (2002) offers a rich elaboration of alongsideness in relation to her work as a health visitor.

6 *Quiet leaders promote self-organised team working*. In their patterns of working and communication, quiet leaders convey a message to others, namely, 'We can do it ourselves'. This strengthens and encourages everyone. They believe that members of the team are capable of making safe and principled decisions about their work. A self-organising spirit works best with teams with a strong culture of care and where the practices of reflection are part of everyone's professional disposition. This culture helps members self-regulate (Schunk & Zimmerman 1998), adjust, revise and accommodate. The quiet leader is in the role of 'steward'.

7 *Quiet leaders are not thick-but thin-skinned*. Quiet leaders are emotionally literate ones. They stay tuned-in to how the team is feeling. They are aware of the emotions within the team and are sensitive to the teams 'emotional labours' (Henderson 2001). This kind of labouring calls for a coordination of mind and feeling that helps to create, in others, a sense of being cared for in a convivial and safe place. But quiet leaders display emotions that are not just professional and polite, but genuine. Their thinness of skin also enables them to work effectively at the interface between emotion and learning (Antonacopoulou & Gabriel 2001). This again is apparent in the story of Dot and particularly her cognisance of the subtleties between emotion at the individual and team level and what helps or inhibits team working and learning.

8 *Quiet leaders appreciate that little things matter a great deal*. Another way of expressing this is that they appear to work with an awareness of the 'butterfly effect'. In the 1960s the modern study of chaos began with an appreciation that tiny differences in input to a system could quickly become large differences in output. This phenomenon was called a 'sensitive dependence on initial conditions' (Gleick 1991). The butterfly effect was an idea that a butterfly stirring the air in Peking today, could transform storm systems next month in New York. The idea is highly relevant in healthcare as we endeavour to think more collectively and systemically in a world of service modernisation that is highly connected and interdependent. Quiet leaders appear to be aware of this butterfly effect. I have observed this in their attention to the 'little things'; a quiet and encouraging word to a member of staff,

which lifts the head and heart for the rest of the day and breathes renewed life into her/his work with patients. I have heard this as they express their concern that 'little things do matter'. I have seen it at work in team meetings when there is a strong commitment to 'sorting things out here' and getting it right locally. A patient enters a clinic for an appointment and from this moment everything that follows is sensitively dependent upon this initial encounter, the initial conditions.

9   *Quiet leaders are resistant to the responsibility virus.* Quiet leaders seem to have a natural predisposition to avoid mishandling responsibility. The responsibility virus (Martin 2003) sets up leaders (and followers) for failure. There are two aspects to the virus, over-responsibility and under-responsibility. Martin (2003, p. 8) puts it like this: '... *it is human nature to claim credit when things go well and to avoid blame when they go badly ... These are the inner drives that push us to the extremes of over-responsibility and under-responsibility ... The virus propels the heroic leader to a failure generated by taking on more responsibility than any one person can carry. But then, as over-responsible leaders approach the point of failure, they do an abrupt turnaround, flipping to an under-responsible stance in order to insulate themselves from the pain and responsibility they see looming'.* This vacillation between over and under-responsibility can be an endless, degenerating experience. Quiet leaders seem to work out ways to inoculate themselves and others against this virus.

10   *Quiet leaders have a quality of mystique.* This is a defining attribute. Quiet leaders act quietly. This does not mean silently (de Vries 2001). Quiet leaders are not the high profile, most senior, visible and 'noisy' public figures within organisations. They work patiently, carefully, incrementally, almost inconspicuously over time (Collins 2001). They work with modesty and restraint and do not seek the spotlight. They work within teams and see teams as the new power house for modernisation. I have found them working in unglamorous, ordinary, person-centred ways, almost invisible and often unnoticed by those outside and above. Their careful, small and practical efforts are what really makes a difference to the quality of team member's working life and to services. They have an abundance of 'soft skills'. All of this just adds to their mystique.

A serious question is: Why are some highly successful leaders also very self-effacing, modest and eager to share credit? Perhaps this is because:

- Humility gives others in the team space to flourish.
- Team success depends upon staff having a sense of ownership of the team's improvement process.
- They understand how important it is for staff to feel valued.
- They appreciate that their views are not always necessarily right.
- They know that being wrong does not mean feeling diminished.
- They embrace the fact that becoming a leader is always 'work in progress'.

Creativity, coping with work and recovery

This is a complex interplay of capacities and capabilities within the creative zone. Being creative requires a sense of purpose and perseverance, courage and conviction. These are all potentially energy sapping. Team members need to balance a commitment to 'being creative' with adequate self-care. A collective 'must-do' is reflecting on ways to rest and rejuvenate and to reconnect with the values the team finds inspiring and meaningful. A serious interest for reflective teams becomes a creative exploration of maximising performance by alternating periods of activity with periods of rest and recovery. Developing reflective teams is therefore about reflecting on 'work-rest ratios'. Through **TA²LK**, staff are encouraged to explore this by discussing how thinking and acting differently is dependent upon supportive work-rest ratios within the team.

The expression 24/7 describes a world in which work never ends. For some, their experience of working in the NHS is that of working in a world hostile to rest. There is no resting time. Working in such cultures, and at a feverish pace, may even become addictive. So we begin to resist precisely those things that make us more effective. These are taking breaks, seeking restoration and protecting our recovery time. What compounds the problem is that in some healthcare organisations, workaholics are admired, encouraged and financially rewarded. The flipside is that those staff who describe themselves as workaholics have a significantly higher than average incidence of alcohol abuse, divorce and stress-related illnesses! Coping with work, perceptions of work pressure, being workaholics and overworking all affect our capacity to be creative. Additionally, leadership and decision-making within the team all have performance consequences. Some consequences lead to sickness, anxiety, negativity, anger, a lack of concentration and a loss of passion for our work. Others can be inspirational and renewing. Thinking and acting differently, with an improvement purpose in mind, is difficult. The status quo seems to have a magnetic pull on us. Full engagement in the creative process (Loehr & Schwartz 2005) requires staff to reflect on ways to cultivate a dynamic balance between their expenditure and renewal of energy.

Specifically this is reflecting upon ways a team is:

- physically energised;
- emotionally connected;
- mentally focussed; and
- spiritually aligned with a purpose beyond their immediate self-interest (Loehr & Schwartz 2005, p. 5).

Chapter 24

The Service Improvement Zone: making a difference

The 'care zone' focused on *emotional literacy*, and the 'creative zone' on *realistic optimism*. The 'service improvement zone' focuses on *making a difference* to health service practice and policy. The impact of this is often predicated on the nature of development in the other zones. Development in this zone is about the team's ability to manage their impact, skilfully. Reflection and developmental action is in two broad areas. These are shown in Table 24.1.

In developing a team's ability to reflect-for-improvement, it is important to clarify that the purpose of reflection is not necessarily to be the best, to develop a strategy to be the best, a plan to be the best. The purpose of engaging in the practices of reflection may be to develop an understanding of what a team feels they can be the best at. This distinction is absolutely crucial (Collins 2001).

Sustainable service improvement is a complex process involving:

- *Strategy*. A practical and positive plan to make a difference.
- *Tactics*. Adapting the plan 'on the spot' to cope with unforeseen circumstances.
- *Logistics*. Making sure staff have the resources they need when they are required.

In the **TA²LK** process the role of the facilitator (either internal or external to the team) is crucial when staff focus on making a difference. This is the moment when earlier conversations of possibility turn into concrete plans for action. In this zone, some of the most common reflective conversations are about:

- *Avoiding imprudent action.* For some staff, it is not that they cannot or refuse to act (to change) but they act hastily, without direction or imprudently.
- *Developing contingency plans.* This helps team members respond to a natural worry: What will we do if our plan for positive change is not working? Contingency plans help staff become more effective tacticians.
- *Overcoming procrastination.* Facilitators have to work with those who keep putting action off with reasons or excuses. Sometimes staff are very active and full of good ideas, but when it comes to the crunch, they avoid taking the most important steps or making the critical

Table 24.1   Attributes of the service improvement zone.

Attribute	Description
Innovation	The extent to which you feel you can 'try things out' and be creative in your work. *Sample item: I can suggest, to others, ways to improve what we do.*
Influence	The extent to which you feel collectively involved in shaping and developing your service. *Sample item: I really feel we are able to make a difference in our work.*

decisions. They begin to talk themselves out of the very things they said they were committed to doing!

- *Finding incentives and rewards.* These may change as staff go through the process of planning for positive change and then working towards this. Sustained actions need to be rewarded in some way.

Sometimes teams are unable to become innovative in their practice and unable to shape and develop policies that influence service delivery. There are many reasons why this happens. In the **TA²LK** process, there is a clear transition state where, in planning for positive change (see Table 24.2), staff move from feeling relatively comfortable to feeling more vulnerable. This part of the team's development can be very anxiety provoking. An illustration of this follows.

A lived scenario: going somewhere or nowhere?

A group of 10 health visitors are engaging in **TA²LK**. This is their third session. The previous two have been well attended. Six manage to attend for this two-hour meeting, 9.30 to 11.30 a.m. Their line manager has not attended any of the sessions. Two facilitators, external to the team, have been working with them.

The planned purpose of the session is to collectively draft a positive (action) plan for change. Staff are keen to develop better practice to reduce the effects of passive smoking in children and particularly very young ones. They are aware that 42% of children in their locality live in households where someone smokes. They want to use some of the session to explore options for risk reduction, at home. Time goes quickly. By 11.00 a.m. the group are deep in conversation about how passive smoking harms family life, about coughs and colds, middle ear infections and asthma. There are rich conversations about children living in smoky homes, smoky rooms, improved ventilation and smoke-free areas.

Then everything stops. Turning the conversations into a positive plan for change seems like a huge task. Paralysis sets in. Nobody can make the first move. They are not sure what they can put on paper. They agree to do nothing. The reason they give is that they cannot speak for other group members who are not present.

Some of the following influences on (in)action are relevant to understanding this scenario.

Facilitators without an action mentality

This is when facilitators respond to the passivity (in-action) of staff with a kind of passivity of their own. For example, responding with comments like, 'Well it's up to you!'. To avoid this, facilitators need to enable participants to be active in the reflective sessions, own as much of the process as possible and help appreciate the need for action.

Staff inertia

Some participants put off the moment to make a decision, to get started, to take the first step. There are many reasons why participants may avoid taking this responsibility. Some common ones are:

- *Passivity.* Not acting in situations that need action. This includes doing nothing, uncritically accepting goals and suggestions made by others, becoming paralysed to act or even becoming aggressive (shutting down or letting off steam).
- *Learned helplessness.* This helplessness means staff can do nothing to change/improve the situation. There are 'degrees' of helplessness, such as 'I'm not up to this' to feelings of deep inadequacy often coupled with a depressive state. Facilitators need to enable participants to know what is and is not in their control.
- *Disabling self-talk.* This is where team members talk themselves out of things and into passivity. Conversations slide into problems, obstacles, 'It won't work' and 'We can't do it'. Facilitators have to get staff to confront this.
- *Vicious cycles.* When plans don't go well and with knock backs, staff can lose a sense of self-worth, lose heart and confidence in their plan for change. This can spiral a team downwards into a mindset of defeat and depression. Staff need to reflect on the entire improvement cycle and appreciate that sometimes things get worse before they get better. Celebrating small successes can be the start of a 'virtuous cycle'.

Table 24.2   Planning for positive change.

In summary, our single PRIORITY FOR ACTION is …
What we have AGREED to do FIRST is …
ONE ANTICIPATED DIFFICULTY is …
Our PLAN to MANAGE this is …
We think EVIDENCE of POSITIVE CHANGE will be …

Feeling that things are falling apart

Sometimes team members have a tendency to give up on action they have initiated. Some action to implement a positive plan for change can begin strongly but then dwindle and stop. Plans seem realistic, achievable and begin with enthusiasm. Then their implementation becomes tedious. What seemed easy at the start now seems to be quite difficult. Participants flounder, get discouraged and may give up.

Choosing not to change

Some staff develop new understandings and awareness, of themselves and others, their work and workplaces. They even appreciate what they need to do to change the current situation. But they choose not to act. They do not want to 'pay the price' called for by fully committing to the action. Facilitators need to help participants understand the consequences of not changing. But in the end it is the participant's choice not to act.

In developing as a reflective team, staff are encouraged to secure a workable level of agreement with regard to the statements in Table 24.2.

Chapter 25

Evidence of positive change and sustainable improvement

TA²LK is an evidence-generating process. Evidence is more than personal anecdote, impression or feeling. Evidence can be used by staff to support claims they make that **TA²LK** has (or has not) helped them make a difference. **TA²LK** helps generate (at least) four forms of evidence. They are:

- *Spoken.* Staff testimony.
- *Written.* Each team is given a **TA²LK** booklet in which to record the outcomes of their reflective conversations.
- *Pictoral.* Graphical.
- *Numerical.* Statistical analysis of questionnaire data.

What evidence is gathered and with what purpose in mind is a matter of judgement from members of the team involved. Evidence can be used in many ways, for example to influence, convince, persuade, support, justify and benchmark. Reflective conversations about evidence for real service improvement often begin with:

1 What evidence do we need?
2 How much do we collect?
3 What do we do with it, when we've got it?

Not all change is an improvement. Not all improvement can be sustained. Many reflective conversations are usually needed for staff to be sure that their positive plan for change has matured into some kind of sustainable improvement in practice or policy. Some common concerns raised by teams during this process, with some questions to stimulate further team reflection, are shown in Table 25.1.

In the team's **TA²LK** booklet staff are encouraged to record the outcomes of their reflective conversations, about sustainable improvement, in a 'brief-but-vivid' manner. The catalysts for thinking are:

1 In summary, the improvement made is …
2 The evidence to support this claim is …
3 Our plan to keep this improvement going is …
4 Our plan to keep this improvement visible to others is …

TA²LK and benchmarking

This process of developing reflective healthcare teams that are able to sustain high quality, personalised care, makes learning visible for all

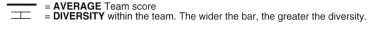

──── = **AVERAGE** Team score
⊥ = **DIVERSITY** within the team. The wider the bar, the greater the diversity.

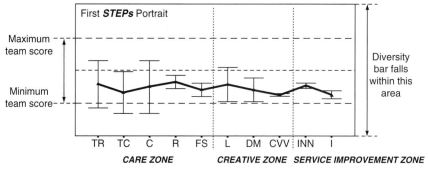

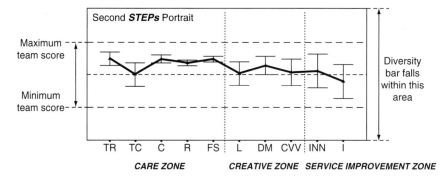

Fig 25.1   STEPs... and benchmarking progress.

participants. A further example of this is when staff repeat the use of STEPs (and/or SURE) over time. The first STEPs portrait acts as a benchmark. Then there is an intervening period when staff formulate, implement and evaluate, the impact of their positive plan for change on services and/or policy. Staff decide when to repeat the completion of the second STEPs questionnaire. The first and second portraits are then compared. This can be done visually. They act as catalysts for further reflective conversations (see Fig. 25.1).

Statistical analyses can also be provided for teams to determine 'significant' improvements (or otherwise) over time. This benchmarking process, within **TA²LK**, is a way teams get a real sense of their own development and the development of services. Figure 25.1 shows a marked improvement in well-being between STEPs 1 and 2 (14 months) for this team. The second STEPs portrait depicts a much healthier team. Improvements have been made across all ten attributes. The depressed team line and corrosive degree of diversity initially, within the team's care zone, has been significantly reduced. They are beginning to feel like a 'proper team', although more conversations need to be devoted to team

Table 25.1 Moving towards evidence-based sustainable improvement.

Concern	Reflective Questions
We don't have enough evidence.	How far do you think you can get very big messages from small amounts of evidence?
We have too much evidence.	How far can you discriminate between what's useful or probably not?
The evidence is not good enough.	So what's the best thing to do now?
We don't want to listen to our evidence.	How far is it telling you something that's too painful for you to cope with right now?
We cannot understand the evidence.	How are you looking at and listening to it?
We need to match the evidence with the audience.	How do you plan to communicate what you know to others?
We need to present our evidence clearly.	How can you present it to be persuasive and influence decisions?

cohesion. There are clear signs that the team is becoming more emotionally literate and developing a good sense of optimism. When treated diagnostically, these portraits enable teams to use their energies (physical, mental, emotional and spiritual) in a much more targeted and effective manner. Currently this team is devising another positive plan for change to tackle issues that are now surfacing with regard to becoming more innovative and influential in their practice.

Managing the improvement process is a very skilful business. Teams have to be in good health to do this. There are always things that will help teams and get in the way. When things begin to change there are often intended effects and unintentional consequences. As a team's improvement effort gains momentum it may spread positively to other teams or be (increasingly) resisted by them. With every improvement process, staff need to manage both the spread effects (positives/benefits) and backwash effects (negatives/difficulties).

Chapter 26

Service user initiated team development

Reflective teams are not only developed 'from within' by working with staff initiated (professional-first) concerns. External influences play an important part also. Increasingly significant sources of external influences are service users and the more general shift to greater patient and public involvement in healthcare. Part of **TA²LK** embraces the significant shift in UK health service delivery which tries to understand the nature and quality of care 'through the patient's eyes'. SURE is a practical contribution to enabling services to be even more patient-centred. In this sense it symbolises New Labour's 'politics of participation'. SURE helps teams reflect on what matters most, and to whom. It systematically and sensitively invites users (anonymously) to share experiences regarding specific 'episodes of care' after all relevant and appropriate 'clearances' and approvals have been secured. There are both advantages and challenges with inviting users to comment on services they are still accessing. SURE provides an opportunity for staff to understand user views, as they continue through their care pathways and on their 'journey' accessing different services as they go. Some teams begin to engage in the **TA²LK** process by eliciting user experiences first. Other teams begin by using STEPs. Choices have to be made and decisions justified.

Briefly, SURE is a retrospective, knowledge-generating process usually done in a number of ways: by service users completing the SURE questionnaire unaided and by themselves with the help of a specially trained **TA²LK** facilitator working 'alongside' them or with a **TA²LK** facilitator going through the statements verbally with the user and recording their responses. Completed questionnaires can be returned via a stamped addressed envelope provided, or placed in special posting boxes in agreed locations within participating organisations. SURE is not an empty ritual. It takes user participation seriously. It is another expression of a shift in the balance of power (DoH 2002) and places user's experiences 'front and central'. As with all other components of **TA²LK**, the essence of it is to provide participants with a way of reflecting systematically, rigorously, creatively, and with hope, on the quality of services in particular settings. It is another dimension of developing reflective teams.

Physio ... therapy through TA²LK

A group of 12 physiotherapists, working in a spinal injuries unit, wanted to have a deeper understanding of the experiences of their patients 'when they came to them'. Through discussion with the team, one particular 'episode' they all wanted to reflect upon was the experiences of patients as they made their transition from their acute into their rehabilitation phase, within the unit. It was decided that, with the patient's full consent, 10 patients making their first outpatient visit, would be invited to re-spond to the statements in SURE. This occurred, with four patients completing it with assistance from a fully trained **TA²LK** facilitator. The idea was that the SURE portrait would be looked at and discussed, by the team, in a number of their 'peer support' meetings. It was regarded as a catalyst for possibly thinking and acting differently. This was done. The first portrait is shown in Fig. 26.1.

Figure 26.1 shows that SURE portraits are fed back to participants in a format, similar to STEPs portraits. They are again made up of two messages. One is reflected by the solid (wavy) line, the other by a bar of different widths. What is different is that the line and bars refer to 10 'experiential areas'. But like STEPs, these are grouped into three zones. Again, this portrait is a catalyst for a conversation of possibility. Different versions of SURE are used with different services in mind (e.g. maternity, children's services). The reflections of this user group show a high level of vulnerability and relatively low scores around patient choice, privacy and dignity, support from staff and involvement. The varying width of the bar, around each point, was a fertile area for team reflection and future action. Different SUREs are available for different services.

The physiotherapy team made and implemented a plan for action. The team's plan concentrated on issues of 'communication' and how this related to 'patient vulnerability'. Through a series of reflective conversa-tions, the team began to talk about what they called their 'core principles', which they believed should underpin all professional, patient and carer communications. *Understandability* and *timeliness* were regarded as two important core principles. In other words the team reflected upon what they customarily said to their patients and when, as they moved into rehabilitation. *Consistency* also emerged as a core principle. The team were aware (and patients and carers confirmed this) that vulnerability was related to 'being told different things by different staff', a perception of being told different things by junior and more senior staff as well as different messages from staff in different disciplines. Staff explored the possibility that their patients' feelings of vulnerability were linked with issues of support and patients' wanting to 'get back to where they were before'. Additionally, they began to develop their appreciation that there is always the possibility that what patients' hear is not what is said to them.

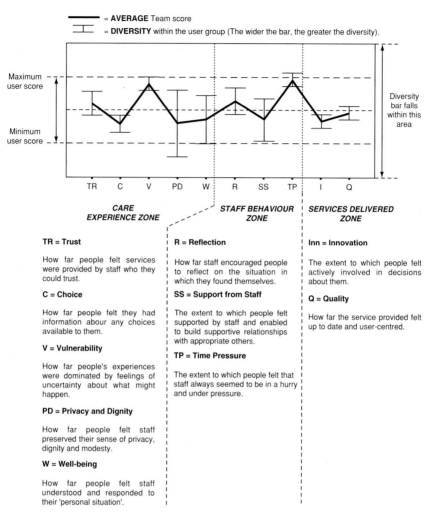

Fig 26.1 Learning from you.

They needed to be open to the fact that what they thought they said, may not always be what they actually said!

The issue of consistency also involved conversations with other disciplines. The physiotherapists had a series, of what they felt were productive meetings, with the unit's team of occupational therapists. Fixing up and having a conversation with some of the nursing and medical staff was more problematic, for reasons I discussed in Part Three. The physiotherapists have sustained a form of *disciplined action*. This raises two points. First, developing reflective teams requires commitment, effort and resources. Second, the interface of team-with-team is a potential site for issues of power, knowledge creation, micro-politics, truth and hope to emerge. It requires another effort. This is where 'communities-of-learners' are extended and real multi-professional learning develops. Six months later another group of ten outpatients were invited to complete SURE. This second portrait was also fed back to the team. In this way team learning and service improvement were fuelled by an iterative process of reflection-with-action.

Chapter 27

Why not try this?

In a part of the TA^2LK process called, 'Why not try this?' staff find a range of team learning and working activities. One particular development activity helps teams decide where they want to focus their attention and energy first. Some teams say, 'I think we'll start by sorting ourselves out, then we'll see what our patient's/clients say'. Other teams say, 'We think we're OK as a team, but we want to check this out with our patients/clients, and go from there'. Generally, those teams with more developed emotional literacies opt for starting with SURE.

What follows is an illustration of one 'orienting' and 'focusing' activity for staff. It serves to make the point that TA^2LK is essentially *about* and *for* the development of practice. In this example, staff comprised a large team of school nurses. This was their first TA^2LK session. Two external facilitators worked with them. The 'post-it' activity unfurls thus:

- Organise yourselves into groups of up to six people.
- Take a moment to privately reflect on what you do.
- Try to focus on one thing, in your work, that really *satisfies* you.
- Write this clearly on your yellow post-it.
- Now focus on one thing, in your work, that *concerns* you.
- Write this clearly on your grey post-it.

Some examples of staff responses are shown in Fig. 27.1.

The activity continues:

- In your group, collect all the yellow and grey post-its together. Then pass them on to another group.
- Look at your new group of yellow and grey post-its. Spend some time reading through each one carefully. As a group, choose one yellow and one grey post-it that you feel able to relate to. Be prepared to say something about your choices.
- Bring your yellow and grey post-its to the main table and stick them down on the large coloured paper provided.

Figure 27.2 shows the post-its that were chosen to be the focus for a whole team conversation about practice.

The 'conversation of possibility' lasted for an hour. On balance, and unsurprisingly, more attention was given to concerns about work rather than satisfactions with work. There were three main themes within the conversation, with connections between them. The themes provided

YELLOW POST-IT RESULTS

- Working with young people and getting positive feedback - Health Education
- Finding a failed hearing test, following it up and getting results
- Being able to help child/family - Responses from children/colleagues
- Meeting a variety of people
- Hearing testing, height and weight screening - Working on own
- BCGs (Don't kill me!)
- Working in a team
- Referral to ENT from our hearing clinics
- Hearing tests
- Working with a variety of different agencies
- Development of the school nurse role from task orientated to child and family focus
- Coming together as a team to do the immunisation

GREY POST-IT RESULTS

- Amount of time spent on paperwork taking us away from parent or child contact
- Occasional barriers put up by teachers which can hinder our work
- Mandatory training updates
- I don't like going into schools and feeling in the way. Unimportant
- Lack of staff and support-Caseloads left vacant... feel that we let schools and children down
- Records missing from clinic
- Missing notes/Records
- What part school nurse assistants will have with the changes
- Communication problems with other agencies
- Lack of recognition of the role in relation to clerical support
- When clients don't attend appointments
- Paperwork

Fig 27.1   The post-it activity: orienting and focusing staff attention.

many ideas for the eventual co-construction of their positive plan for change.

1   *Workload and work overload.* Staff explored what they meant when they talked about 'workload' and 'overload'. This embraced such things as 'the amount of time they felt they had to do things', 'conflicting demands on their time', 'the quantity of work they felt expected to do', 'stress' and 'missing breaks trying to get work done'. An important distinction emerged. Workload was beginning to be seen as

YELLOW POST-IT RESULTS

- Getting to know pupils and helping with their concerns
- The support of work colleagues
- Healthy and happy children
- Working with children and families, enabling them to effect changes

GREY POST-IT RESULTS

- Time constraints - prioritising and re-prioritising and never winning!
- Increasing amount of paperwork - deskbound waste of skills
- Feeling I am not really in control any more with all the changes
- Rushing around, chasing my tail, getting exhausted and not feeling I've achieved anything

Fig 27.2   The post-it activity: building consensus.

'something you can increase or decrease'. Overload was linked with 'simultaneous demands, responsibility and feeling out of control'.

2 *Effort-reward (im)balance.* The school nurses talked passionately about they way having access to information, feeling supported in their job by others in the team, positive feedback from families and schools, career opportunities and working term-time only, affected their perception of effort-reward (im)balance. The degree of flexibility, their ability to exercise their judgement and job meaning were all discussed. What began to emerge was a sense that better team working and learning might play some kind of protective role in reducing the likelihood of effort-reward imbalance.

3 *Balancing a commitment to others with adequate self-care.* The team explored how they might balance their desire to 'provide a good service' and maximise their performance, without feeling constantly drained and burnt out. They mentioned things like praise and thanks, helping children and guiding families, optimism, dedication and encouragement. They were alluding to aspects of emotional literacy.

This team decided that their next move would be to learn through STEPs. Their eventual plan for positive action was: How we can get even more satisfaction from our work.

Chapter 28

Developing reflective teams: perception and reality

One way we deceive ourselves is by assuming that our view represents the truth, when it is actually just an interpretation. We all use different lenses to view the world. Sometimes, almost without realising it, we create stories around a set of experiences and then take this to be the truth on the matter. **TA²LK** develops teams by enabling staff to see how far a 'good team translates into a good service'. A comparison of STEPS and SURE portraits is a way they can do this. It opens up the possibility for a different kind of conversation amongst staff. Teams often require healthy levels of emotional literacy and realistic optimism to get the most from this process. Staff may have to retain an ongoing openness to the possibility that they may not be seeing themselves, or others, accurately. Sometimes staff say with incredulity: Is that us? Is that how they really see us? Although on occasions it can be difficult and unpleasant, when comparisons are made between staff and user views of services, we know at least two things can change. First, a team's learning trajectory can change. Second, a team's rate of development alters. A sign of a developing team is their 'Janusian ability' to look outwards and to learn from service user experiences, their local health economy and the 'system', and inwards to learn from the gifts and talents, hopes and anxieties of each member of the team.

Emotionally literate and realistically optimistic teams have this Janusian quality. They have an openness and receptivity about them. Often they keep moving forward because they are sufficiently 'healthy' and well developed to recognise that the forces of self-protection slow up the service improvement process. They are aware that self-protection can escalate into self-sealing team processes and that these seriously hinder team development. Their level of well-being means that successes, however small, are noticed and celebrated. Because all change requires moving beyond our comfort zone, it is best initiated and sustained in small manageable steps. Teams that are realistically optimistic are far more likely to experience success, because each step they make is a small one.

Developing reflective teams that are able to sustain high quality, personalised care

During the period 1999–2004 a data base of work with 753 teams in health and social care in the UK and 3211 service users has been gathered. These

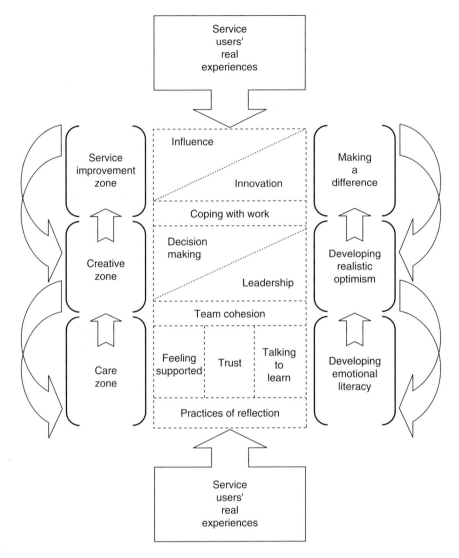

Fig 28.1 A generic and holistic model for developing the reflective healthcare team through TA²LK.

data, and their qualitative and quantitative (regression) analyses, provide the basis for the generic and holistic model shown in Fig. 28.1. It is a model that depicts a way of developing reflective teams that are able to sustain high quality, personalised care. It is grounded in evidence 'from the field' and overcomes the limitations of earlier linear, one-way or 'stage' team development models. It focuses on much more than team roles, however flexible.

The essence of the model is this

1 Its *focus is on team learning*, facilitated through the interests and practices of reflection. It links team development with the team's ability to learn. It makes *learning and development visible* to all those involved.

2 It is underpinned by forms of *disciplined and supported reflection-and-action*, which enable teams to sustain high quality, personalised care.

3 *It emphasises learning through sharing*. This process influences a team's wellness and general health. Wellness affects how far teams are able to influence change and respond positively to it.

4 It views the development of reflective teams as a social process supported within *inclusive communities of participation*. These communities need to be understood as patterns of action and interaction.

5 *It rejects team development as a linear process*. It is more complex than this. There is not one team development trajectory. Teams move back and forth presenting and then discarding 'faces' according to the exigencies of the moment.

6 It describes the genesis and attributes of *three fundamental team 'faces'*. These are the: (*a*) face of the *emotionally literate* team; (*b*) face of teams that are *realistically optimistic*; and (*c*) face of teams that *make a difference*.

7 *Changing faces* is accepted as normal and responsive to service demands and policy imperatives. Each change creates new team learning opportunities. These *are catalysts for further conversations of possibility*. Talking to learn is an essential part of developing a reflective team.

8 It helps focus team member's attention and resources on matters significant to them and those they work with and care for. Teams *use their energies* (physical, mental, emotional and spiritual) *in a targeted and strategic manner*.

Reflective teams as sites of struggle

Improving team learning through the interests and practices of reflection, is never done on a flat playing field. Teams develop in different ways. TA^{2}LK allows teams to understand 'where they are at'. It makes learning and development visible. There is no magic, quick fix, express trajectory to better team learning. In general it is a struggle. A bumpy, up-and-down process. Clearly talking to learn is an essential part of developing a reflective team. Teams who engage in TA^{2}LK create a space in their professional lives for regeneration and for learning through the interests and practices of reflection. This space can be the site where issues of power, politics, truth and hope emerge. It is a space where knowledge for service improvement and workplace transformation can be integrated.

In undertaking work for this book, I have learnt that there are at least three pervasive kinds of struggle for teams. First, the struggle against *domination* (e.g. from more powerful individuals, teams, disciplines). Second, the struggle against *exploitation* (e.g. being locked into a one-way street of giving and serving others and never receiving). Third, the struggle against *de-professionalisation* (e.g. due to being unable to defend one's corner in the light of moves to re-design workforces, visions of a new work order and therefore new work cultures).

The book's central question is: How can we develop reflective healthcare teams that are able to sustain high quality, personalised care? In summary, I hope Fig. 28.1 describes an evidence-based way to do this. There is now sufficient evidence to suggest that these teams are a vibrant resource for struggle, giving staff and service users, energy, courage and a *collective creative consciousness* to improve services and workplaces. I have learnt that reflective teams are a source for being-human-well *and* a resource for struggle. This is why, I believe, they are worth developing. What is your view?

References

Antonacopoulou, E.P. & Gabriel, Y. (2001) Emotion, learning and organizational change. *Journal of Organizational Change Management* **14**(5), 435–451.

Ashforth, B. & Humphrey, R. (1995) Emotion in the workplace: a reappraisal. *Human Relations* **48**(2), 97–124.

Ashkanasy, N., Zerbe, W. & Hartel, C. (eds) 2002. *Managing Emotions in the Workplace*. M.E. Sharpe, New York.

Bar-On, R., Brown, J. Kirkcaldy, B. & Thome, E. (2000) Emotional expression and implications for occupational stress: an application of the emotional quotient inventory (EQ-I). *Personality and Individual Differences* **28**, 1107–118.

Belbin, M. (1982) *Management Teams: Why They Succeed or Fail*. Heinemann, London.

Bennis, W. (1993) *An Invented Life: Reflections on Leadership and Change*. Addison-Wesley, Reading, Massachusetts.

Burbules, N. (1993) *Dialogue in Teaching: Theory and Practice*. Teacher's College Press, New York.

Bernhard, L.A. & Walsh, M. (1995). *Leadership: The Key to the Professionalization of Nursing*, 3rd edn. Mosby, St Louis.

Cherniss, C. & Goleman, D. (eds) (2001) *The Emotionally Intelligent Workplace*. Jossey-Bass, San Fransisco.

Collins, J. (2001) *Good to be Great: Why Some Companies Make the Leap … and Others Don't*. Harper Business, New York.

Costa, A.C., Roe, R.A. & Taillieu, T. (2001) Trust within teams: the relation with performance effectiveness. *European Journal of Work and Organizational Psychology* **10**(3), 225–244.

Daly, J. (1993) Overcoming the barrier of words. In *Through the Patients Eyes* (eds M. Gerteis, S. Edgman-Levitan, J. Daly & T.L. Delbanco). Jossey Bass, San Francisco.

Department of Health (2002) *Shifting the Balance of Power: The Next Steps*. DoH, London.

DePree, M. (1997) *Leading without Power: Finding Hope in Serving Community*. Jossey-Bass, New York.

de Vries, M. K. (2001) *The Leadership Mystique: A User's Manual for the Human Enterprise*. Pearson Education, Edinburgh.

Donnor, G.J. & Wheeler, M.M. (2004) New strategies for developing leadership. *Nursing Leadership* **17**(2), 27–32.

Durant, R. (2002) Synchronicity: a post-structuralist guide to creativity and change. *Journal of Organizational Change Management* **15**(5), 490–501.

Fairholm, M.R. & Fairholm, G. (2000) Leadership amid the constraints of trust. *Leadership and Organization Development Journal* **21**(2), 102–109.

Fisher, C. & Ashkanasy, N. (2000) The emerging role of emotions in work life: an introduction. *Journal of Organizational Behavior* **21**, 123–129.

Fitzgerald, L., Ferlie, E. & Hawkins, C. (2003) Innovation in healthcare: how does credible evidence influence professionals? *Health and Social Care in the Community* **11**(3), 219–28.

Freire, P. (1972) *The Pedagogy of the Oppressed*. Penguin, Harmondworth.

French, S. (2004) Challenges to developing and providing leadership. *Nursing Leadership* **17**(4), 37–40.

Freshman, B. & Rubino, L. (2002) Emotional intelligence: a core competency for health care administrators. *The Health Care Manager* **20**(4), 1–9.

Gadamer, H. (1979) *Truth and Method*. Sheed and Ward, London.

Gladwell, M. (2002) *The Tipping Point: How Little Things Can Make a Big Difference*. Little, Brown, Boston.

Gleick, J. (1991) *Chaos*. Cardinal Press.

Groesbeck, R. & van Aken, E.M (2001) Enabling team wellness: Monitoring and maintaining teams after start-up. *Team Performance Management* **7**(1/2), 11–20.

Habermas, J. (1984) *The Theory of Communicative Action*, volume 1. Polity Press, Cambridge.

Handy, C. (1996) The new language of organising and its implications for leaders. In *The Leader of the Future* (eds F. Hesselbein *et al.*). Jossey-Bass, San Francisco.

Harré, R. (1983) *Personal Being: A Theory for Individual Psychology*. Blackwell, Oxford.

Harrison, S. (2003) Right a bit more. *Health Matters* **44**.

Henderson, A. (2001) Emotional labour and nursing: an under-appreciated aspect of caring work. *Nursing Inquiry* **8**(2), 130–138.

Herbert, R. & Edgar, L. (2004) Emotional intelligence: a primal dimension of nursing leadership? *Nursing Leadership* **17**(4), 56–63.

Hunt, P. (2003) Curtains for Whitehall farce. *Health Service Journal* **1**.

Institute of Medicine (2001) *Crossing the Quality Chasm: A New Health System for the 21st Century*. National Academy of Sciences Press, Washington.

IRP-UK (2005) *TA²LK: The Essence of Improvement*. The Institute of Reflective Practice, IRP-UK, Gloucester.

Kluska, K.M., Spence Laschinger, H.K. & Kerr, M.S. (2004) Staff nurse empowerment and effort-reward imbalance. *Nursing Leadership* **17**(1), 112–128.

Kur, E. (1996) The faces model of high performing team development. *Management Development Review* **9**(6), 25–35.

Loehr, J. & Schwartz, T. (2005) *The Power of Full Engagement: Managing energy, not Time, is the Key to High Performance and Personal Renewal*. The Free Press, New York.

Lofy, M.M. (1998) The impact of emotion on creativity in organizations. *Empowerment in Organizations* **6**(1), 5–12.

Martin, R.L. (2003) *The Responsibility Virus*. Pearson Education, Edinburgh.

Mayer, J. & Salovey, P. (1993) The intelligence of emotional intelligence. *Intelligence* **17**, 433–442.

O'Connor, C. (1993) Managing resistance to change. *Management Development Review* **6**(4), 25–29.

Ollila, S. (2000) Creativity and innovativeness through reflective project leadership. *Creativity and Innovation Management* **9**(3), 195–200.

Parker, F.M. & Morris, A.H. (2004) Shared decision-making in nursing education. *Nursing Leadership* **17**(3), 41–51.

Pellicer, L.O. (2003) *Caring Enough to Lead*. Corwin Press, California.

Perryman, S. & Robinson, D. (2003) Down the line. *Health Service Journal*, 17 April.

Peter, E. (2004) Commentary: who will define the values? *Nursing Leadership* **17**(3), 28–40.

Pound, R. (2002) *How can I improve my health visiting support of parenting? The creation of an alongside epistemology through action enquiry*. Unpublished PhD, Faculty of Education, University of the West of England.

Richards, J. (2004) Commentary: a call to think differently. *Nursing Leadership* **17**(1), 62–77.

Rogers, W.R. (1995) The psychological contract of trust – part II. *Executive Development* **8**(2), 7–15.

Rust, J., Golombok, S. & Gill, A. (2003) *Orpheus TPQ*. The Psychological Corporation, San Francisco.

Sashkin, M. & Sashkin, M.G. (2003) *Leadership that Matters*. Berrett-Koehler Publishers, San Francisco.

Schunk, D.H. & Zimmerman, B.J. (1998) *Self-Regulated Learning*. The Guilford Press, New York.

Snow, J. (2001) Looking beyond nursing for clues to effective leadership. *Journal of Nursing Administration* **31**(9), 440–443.

Stott, K. & Walker, A. (1995) *Teams, Teamwork and Teambuilding*. Prentice Hall, London.

Syer, J. & Connolly, C. (1996) *How Teamwork Works: the Dynamics of Effective Team Development*. McGraw-Hill, New York.

Tuckman, B.W. (1965) Development sequence in small groups. *Psychological Bulletin* **63**, 384–399.

Vitello-Cicciu, J. (2002) Exploring emotional intelligence: implications for nursing leaders. *Journal of Nursing Administration* **32**(4), 203–210.

Weare, K. (2004) *Developing the Emotionally Literate School*. Paul Chapman.

Weisinger, H. (1998) *Emotional Intelligence at Work*. Jossey-Bass, New York.

Wheatley, M.J. (1999) *Leadership and the New Science*. Berrett-Koehler, San Francisco.

Index